MEDICAL EMERGENCIES

WHAT TO DO FIRST

1. MAKE SURE THE VICTIM IS BREATHING.
2. STOP HEAVY BLEEDING.
3. PREVENT FURTHER INJURY.
4. BE ALERT TO THE SIGNS OF SHOCK.
5. DO NOT ATTEMPT ANY FIRST AID THAT YOU ARE NOT FAMILIAR WITH.
6. ASK SOMEONE TO GET MEDICAL HELP.

WHAT TO TELL THE DOCTOR

1. WHERE IS THE VICTIM?
2. WHAT HAS HAPPENED?
3. WHO IS CALLING?
4. YOUR PHONE NUMBER? ______________
5. WILL EXTRA HELP BE NEEDED?
6. ANY QUESTIONS?

HELP YOURSELF TO SWIFT, AUTHORITATIVE ADVICE . . .

—When your child suddenly starts running a high fever
—When you're faced with a puncture wound spouting blood
—When someone is choking before your very eyes
—When an insect bite produces exaggerated swelling and pain
—When you've burned your hand with scalding liquid

You can't afford to be helpless when such emergencies strike. That's why this book was written—and why you should always have it within easy reach for instant aid.

Emergency Handbook

A FIRST AID MANUAL
FOR HOME AND TRAVEL

ABOUT THE AUTHORS:

PETER ARNOLD is the author of *Checklist for Emergencies.*

EDWARD L. PENDAGAST, JR., M.D., A.C.E.P., is Director of the Emergency Department of New Milford Hospital in Connecticut.

Emergency Handbook

A FIRST AID MANUAL
FOR HOME AND TRAVEL

by Peter Arnold

with Edward L. Pendagast, Jr. M.D.,
Consulting Physician

Illustrations by Charles McVicker

PUBLISHER'S NOTE

The ideas, procedures, and suggestions contained in this book are not intended as a substitute for consulting with your physician. All matters regarding your health require medical supervision.

Doubleday and Company, Inc.,
245 Park Avenue, New York, New York 10017.

This is an authorized reprint of a hardcover edition published by Doubleday and Company, Inc.

2 3 4 5 6 7 8 9

PRINTED IN THE UNITED STATES OF AMERICA

To my new friends,
my dear family
and, especially,
to Jeremy.

ACKNOWLEDGMENTS

MEN AND WOMEN in a great many organizations provided information that has helped make this book possible. I am grateful to staff members of the American Automobile Association, the Automobile Club of Southern California, the American Medical Association, the American National Red Cross, Bio-Health Specialists, Inc., of Boston, the Greater Los Angeles Chapter of the National Safety Council, the Los Angeles County Committee on Affairs of the Aging, the National Safety Council, and the United States Department of Health, Education and Welfare.

I am indebted to my editors, Robert D. Preyer and Marlene K. Connor, who saw the need for this book, envisioned a way to make it most useful, and showed great patience that helped make it a reality. I also thank my literary agent, Max Gartenberg, whose fine efforts brought Bob Preyer and me together.

Lastly, I thank Dr. Edward L. Pendagast, Jr. for the many important suggestions he made while reading the manuscript.

The information in this book is designed to be as accurate and useful as possible. Please understand that its intent is to inform, not advise. The book's purpose is to alert you to various first-aid and emergency situations and to offer generally accepted alternatives for the best response. But particular circumstances and individual victims may require specific actions that are not indicated. That is why it is always best to obtain the advice of an expert.

Peter Arnold
Boston

CONTENTS

INTRODUCTION

THERE ARE MANY definitions of "emergency," ranging from "anything the patient considers an emergency, is an emergency," to the much more dangerous belief that "only disease or injury offering serious threat to life or limb is an emergency." Both ideas are inaccurate and can be costly. However "emergency" is defined, there are millions of visits to the hospital and doctors' offices every year. Many of these visits are unnecessary and waste a great deal of time and money. Many of these emergencies could have been and should have been treated immediately by someone with good, solid knowledge of today's first-aid methods. Very often, the time and physical movement involved in getting an injured or sick person to a hospital emergency room can cause the condition to become *fatal.* This is why it is vital that everyone become familiar with the many life-saving techniques that can be used by the layman. The greater our knowledge of effective first aid, the better everyone's chances will be of surviving a critical injury.

Reading this book will be an important step toward learning the proper procedures for handling many common injuries and illnesses. It is essential, however, that you read and understand it *before* an accident occurs. If it sits on a shelf, you probably won't be able to find it and won't have time to properly use it when a crisis arises. And after reading this book, you might even be stimulated to learn more of today's lifesaving techniques through courses and training classes—which will make the book a real success indeed!

Recent developments in teaching modern first aid, plus the many available courses in CPR (Cardio Pulmonary Resuscitation) from the American Red Cross and the American Heart Association, have made it possible for the trained layman to properly begin treatment for many previously fatal emergencies. In addition, there are thousands of trained rescue personnel available through the Department of Transportation and the Department of Health, Education and Welfare, which are funding courses for police, fire, rescue, and ambulance services, such as the CIM (crash and injury management), EMT (emergency medical technician) the knowledge and skills of these dedicated people have greatly increased the chances of survival for the citizen who is faced with a truly life-threatening emergency.

I hope this book will encourage you to become interested in your local rescue services. Availability and expertise vary from region to region. The need for these rescue services has always been great. What has been lacking is the interest and support of local citizens. An accident doesn't usually happen outside a hospital, where a doctor can be immediately available. Yet proper care should begin at the scene. Without a local rescue team with solid training and up-to-date equipment, many people will suffer needlessly.

If everyone would take the time to understand first aid, it would not be necessary for emergency rooms to be overcrowded with minor bumps, bruises, scrapes, and scratches, or for doctors to have to write orders such as "clean with soap and water" or "apply ice" or "apply Band-Aid." It is even worse to see a patient suffering from a broken bone or ruptured appendix that should have had immediate treatment but didn't because there was no one present who was familiar with any first-aid methods and it took too long to get the victim to the hospital. Over and over, every emergency physician sees cases that graphically demonstrate the need for all to have greater knowledge and more education about themselves and their bodies.

If you will read and use this book, you will have made a healthy beginning step toward basic understanding of first aid. Whether the accident or injury is major or minor, proper care should begin at the scene, by those who are present and by those who respond to a call for help.

There has been a very significant decrease in the death rate from heart attack in communities such as Seattle, Washington, where a concerted community effort has resulted in CPR training of a large proportion of the citizens. Prompt action by a properly trained citizen will often avert tragedy.

The practice of emergency medicine has become progressively more satisfying as more and more of the sick and injured arrive in the emergency department with proper prehospital care. I am seeing much less of the sad cases of my early years in emergency rooms, such as a patient in deep shock or dead from blood loss with no attempt having been made to stop the bleeding, or a coronary dead on arrival without any attempt at CPR, or the stroke victim who died from aspiration for lack of proper positioning. It is essential for everyone to learn the basic skills of first aid and the more advanced skills of CPR if we are going to reduce a death rate that is higher than it ought to be.

Edward L. Pendagast, Jr., M.D.
Director, Emergency Department
New Milford, Conn.

Emergency Handbook

SECTION ONE

Sudden Emergencies

Common but critical situations in which time is a vital factor.

BEE STINGS
(Allergic Reactions)

(Also see Stings by Bees, Wasps and Hornets, pg. 205)

Allergic Reactions

If the victim has an allergic reaction, the simple bee sting can be a serious injury.

Symptoms of allergic reaction include pronounced pain and exaggerated swelling at the sting site, perhaps even extending to large, red, itchy welts (also called hives) on various parts of the body. In extreme cases the patient may suffer from shortness of breath, wheezing, asthma-like respirations, and symptoms of shock (sudden pallor, perspiration, increased pulse rate, decreased blood pressure, perhaps prostration).

Most people who are allergic to bee stings know about their condition. They should *always* carry an emergency bee-sting kit with them when traveling. The kit should contain medication to be taken by mouth and other medication to be injected, including potent antihistamines—which help counteract the venom—and adrenalinlike substances, to combat the shocklike state.

GENERAL PROCEDURE

If an allergic reaction occurs to a person who is unaware of his sensitivity to bee stings, follow this treatment:

- Have the victim lie down. Treat him for shock (see pg. 79).
- Give him whatever antihistamine is carried in the first-aid kit.
- Remove the stinger with an outward scraping motion of the fingernail.

Do *not* pinch the stinger between two fingernails or grasp it with a tweezer, this will cause more venom to spread.

- Apply cold wet dressings to the sting.
- If the allergic reaction is profound—including shortness of breath, wheezing, and shocklike symptoms—send for medical help or get the patient to civilization as soon as possible.
- In most cases, the allergic reaction will subside in 30 minutes.

NOTE: Many more people die from bee stings than from snakebites.

BITES
(Animal)

An animal bite is always serious. The wound is *major* if:

- penetration is beyond the thickness of the skin, or
- the wound is situated on the face, head, or neck, or
- the wound has become infected, or
- the dog, cat, or other animal might have rabies.

NOTE: Bites by *humans* can be major emergencies also. (For treatment, see Scratches pg. 160.)

WHAT TO DO

1. Stop any bleeding.
2. Clean the wound.
3. Cover the wound.
4. Contact a doctor.

Read General Procedure for details.

GENERAL PROCEDURE

- Stop bleeding by applying pressure to area.
- Wash the wound and the surrounding area thoroughly but gently with much warm water and soap. If possible, place the affected area under warm tap water or pour basins of tepid water over the wound (flushing or irrigating the wound).
- Pat it dry with sterile gauze dressing or a clean cloth.
- Apply sterile dressing or an adhesive bandage strip.

- Phone the doctor. Although most people have had their "baby shots," a tetanus booster may be needed to prevent tetanus (lockjaw) caused by contamination. There is also a remote possibility that anti-rabies injections may be needed (a series of 14 shots).
- If the victim has no prior immunization against tetanus, a tetanus antitoxin derived from human volunteers may be administered.

NOTE: Most serious animal bites are by pets that are known to the victims, especially their own or a neighbor's dog. The animal has been startled or has felt threatened. Strange pets and wild animals also inflict bites. Rabies is very rare today, but if the animal is frothing at the mouth, walking erratically, or otherwise acting strange, contact the police. If it must be killed, the head must remain uninjured so that the brain can be examined for rabies. Although human bites do not cause rabies, they are always infected.

A bite wound is *minor* if:

- the skin is only scraped or bruised
- there is no bleeding
- there is no penetration of skin.

GENERAL PROCEDURE

- Clean and disinfect the wound with soap and warm water, preferably holding the affected area under a running faucet.
- Pat the wound dry with sterile dressing or a clean cloth.
- Optional: Apply an antiseptic cream or a detergent cleaner containing benzalkonium (such as Zephiran). But if you've used enough soap with the warm water, this step is not necessary.
- Apply a sterile dressing or a nonsticking adhesive bandage strip (Band-Aid, Curad, etc.).
- Call a doctor. Learn if further treatment is necessary.
- Later, contact the doctor again if:
    1. healing does not progress rapidly, *or*
    2. there is swelling, *or*
    3. there is increased redness or tenderness, *or*
    4. streaks extend outward from the wound.

7

BLEEDING
(External)

Loss of more than one pint of blood is serious. Unchecked bleeding can lead to death. It is essential to control bleeding or hemorrhaging; treat the victim for shock and be alert for cardiac arrest (see Shock, pg. 79 and CPR, pg. 29).

WHAT TO DO

1. Have someone call a hospital ambulance.
2. Apply pressure to the wound.
3. Use a tourniquet only as a last resort.
4. Treat the victim for shock.

Read General Procedure for details

GENERAL PROCEDURE

- If a third person is nearby, have him get professional medical help immediately.
- Place a sterile dressing in the palm of your hand and apply it directly to the wound. If no sterile dressing is available, use a piece of clean cloth. If no clean shirt, towel, handkerchief, or other cloth is within reach, use your hand (washed) to stop the bleeding.
- When the cloth becomes soaked with blood, do *not* remove it. That would increase the blood flow. Instead, apply a new cloth, on top of the old one, with enough pressure to stop the bleeding.
- If the wound is in an arm or leg, raise it to help slow the bleeding. Do *not* raise it if you suspect broken bones.

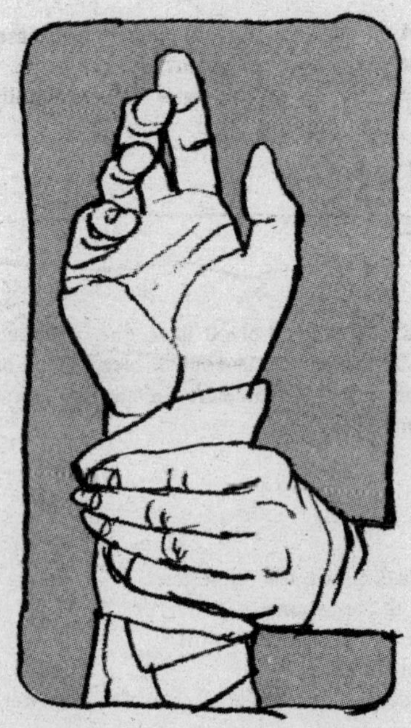

Apply firm pressure.

- If bleeding from an arm or leg continues, keep one hand on the wound and apply the free hand to a pressure point (see illustration). Keep your hand flat as you apply your palm or fingers to the pressure point.

- Give the patient reassurance. Encouragement will ease his fears.
- Use a tourniquet only as a last resort to save a life. For example, use it if a large artery is severed or a limb is wholly or partially severed.

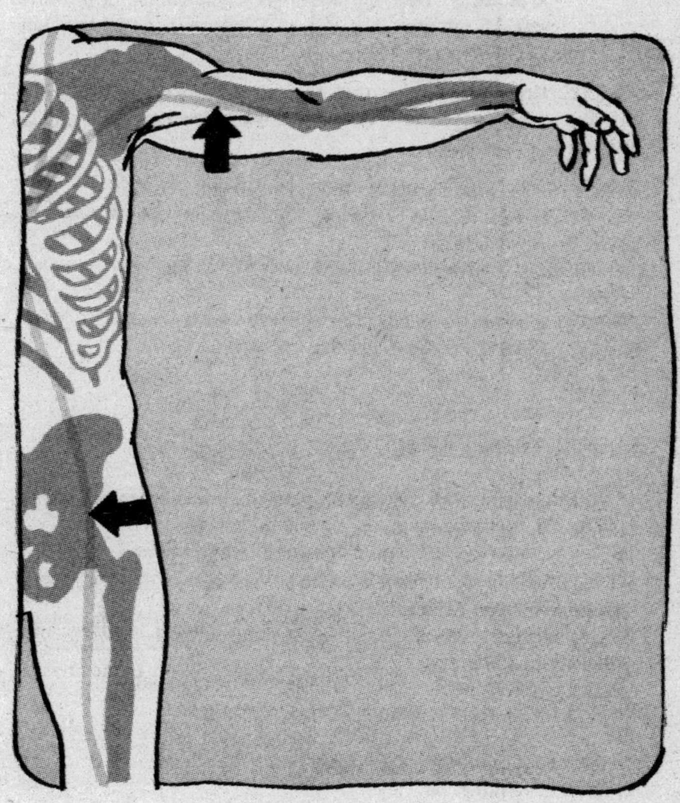

Pressure points.

CAUTION: A tourniquet should be used only as a last resort, to prevent bleeding to death. *Time is important:* the danger is with possible loss of limb due to diminished blood flow. If a hospital is nearby, treat the wound as instructed in General Procedure while rushing the victim to the hospital. If the hospital is too far away, use a tourniquet—briefly releasing the pressure every 15 minutes. The loss of a limb is not as important as loss of life.

NOTE: The Red Cross teaches that once a tourniquet is applied, it is not to be removed. It is best that only medical personnel should apply a tourniquet.

- When the bleeding decreases, tie on the dressing or cloth.
- *Be sure* to treat for shock (see pg. 79). Shock is a major cause of death in accident victims.
- Be prepared to treat cardiac arrest and breathing difficulties (see CPR, pg. 29).

Bleeding is considered *minor* if lost blood in an adult totals no more than one or two ounces and bleeding is controlled fast.

GENERAL PROCEDURE

- Clean and disinfect the wound with soap and warm water, preferably holding the injured area under a running faucet.
- Pat the wound dry with sterile dressing or clean cloth.
- If you like, apply an antiseptic cream or a detergent containing benzalkonium (such as Zephiran).
- Apply a sterile dressing or a nonsticking adhesive bandage strip (Band-Aid, Curad, etc.).
- Call a physician. Learn if medical attention is required.
- Be alert for possible infection. Contact a doctor if

1. the wound does not heal rapidly, *or*
2. there is swelling, *or*
3. there is increased redness or tenderness, *or*
4. streaks extend outward from the wound.

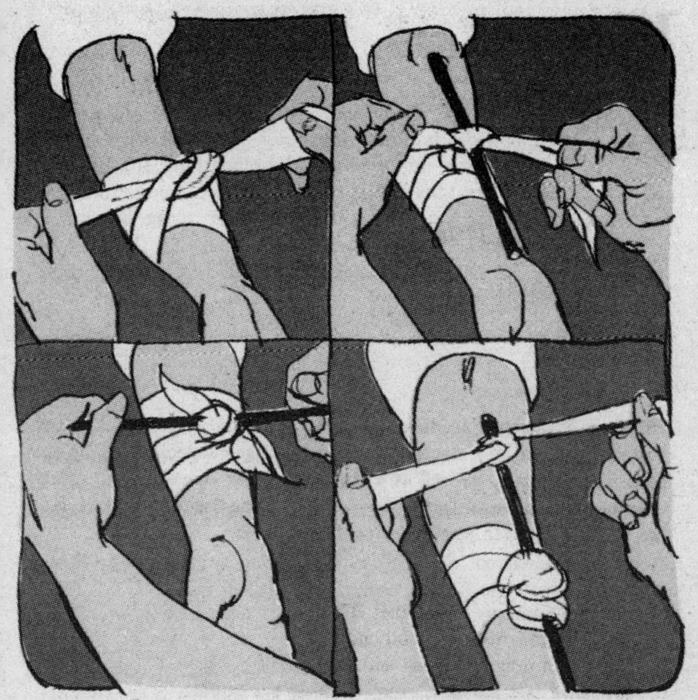

HOW TO TIE A TOURNIQUET

1. *Place a strong, wide piece of cloth (a hankerchief or necktie) close to the wound, between the wound and the heart. Wrap the cloth twice around the arm or leg, then tie a half knot.*

2. *Place a short stick (or ruler) on the half knot, and tie a square knot.*

3. *Twist the stick until all bleeding stops.*

4. *Tie the stick in place with the end of the tourniquet or another piece of cloth, lying the stick flat on the arm or leg and wrapping cloth around.*

12

BLEEDING
(Internal)

All forms of internal bleeding should be considered major unless otherwise determined by a doctor. Internal bleeding can be caused by any hard blow or bump as well as a large number of diseases (e.g., ulcers, cancer). You cannot always recognize bleeding inside the body, and the victim may even appear to feel fine at first.

Signs and Symptoms of Internal Bleeding

1. The skin may be pale, cool, and wet.
2. The victim may feel weak and anxious.
3. The pulse rate is rapid, over 100 beats per minute.
4. There may be vomiting of blood, which may look like ordinary blood or like coffee grounds (which is blood mixed with stomach acid).
5. The victim may be thirsty and ask for water.
6. The victim may have a bloody, black, or tarry bowel movement.

WHAT TO DO

1. Have someone call a hospital ambulance.
2. Make the victim lie down.
3. If there is bleeding from the mouth or nose or the victim becomes unconscious, lay him on his side.
4. If there is trouble breathing, raise the head and shoulders.
5. Check breathing and pulse every 2 to 3 minutes.

6. Give *no* food or drink.
7. Be alert for shock.

Read General Procedure for details.

GENERAL PROCEDURE

- Never allow the victim to walk around. Lay him on his back in a safe, warm place.
- If blood is coming from mouth, or victim is unconscious, *be sure* to place the victim on his *side.*
- Medical help is essential. No first-aid measure will stop internal bleeding. Get medical attention. Surgery and/or a transfusion may be necessary.
- Watch the victim's breathing and pulse rate carefully. If breathing stops, start artificial respiration (see pg. 29).
- *Never* give the victim food or drink.
- Be prepared to treat him for shock.

NOTE: Coughing up pinkish or blood-streaked sputum may be serious, but it is not urgent. Blood from the rectum noted only on the toilet paper and not in the toilet bowl may not be serious. Streaks of blood on the surface of bowel movements also does not usually indicate a dangerous situation. But in all three situations, it is best to *contact a doctor* for an opinion.

14

BONES
(Fractures and Dislocations)

All fractures (also called breaks) and dislocations of large joints are *major* emergencies. If there is a question about the severity of a bone injury, treat it as a fracture or dislocation.

RECOGNIZING THE INJURY

Simple fractures are closed injuries in which the bone remains covered by the skin.

Compound fractures are broken bones plus open wounds leading to the fracture. The most serious breaks occur to the backbone (spine), neck, and pelvis.

Dislocations occur when a bone moves out of its joint. Dislocations often appear to be fractures.

NOTE: Both fractures and dislocations are often accompanied by shock (see pg. 79).

INDICATIONS OF A BROKEN BONE

- A "pop" sound or the victim feels something break.
- Acute tenderness.
- Pain and often swelling.
- Possible deformity.

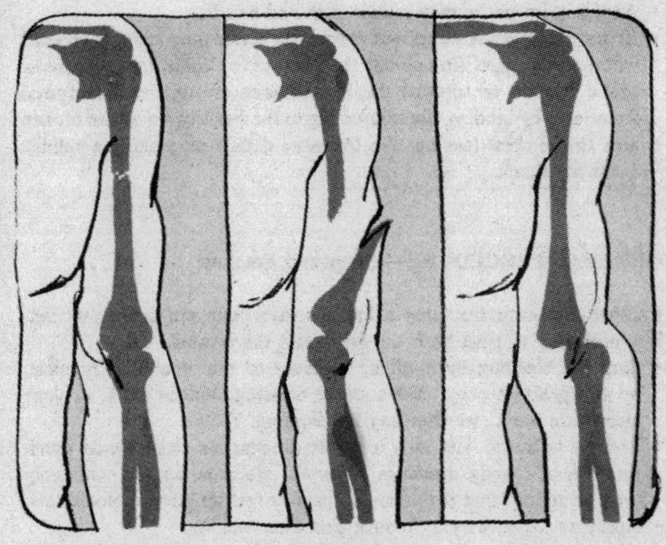

Simple fracture. Compound fracture. Dislocation.

- Partial or complete loss of function.
- Grating sensation upon movement.
- Possible shortening of broken limb.

GENERAL PROCEDURE—Simple Fracture

- *Do not* move the victim unless his present position will result in further harm. Moving will cause pain and possibly further injury.
- *Do not* move the injured area. Do your best to keep the affected area immobile; do not straighten a bent arm or leg.
- Have someone call a hospital ambulance. Do not let the victim of a fractured neck, back, or pelvis sit up or move; using your hands immobilize the head and await an emergency ambulance.

- Applying ice packs may reduce pain and swelling.
- If the victim must be moved before an ambulance arrives, proceed with extreme care. Immobilize the fracture (or limb) *first*, if possible. Make a splint to support the injured area or support the injured leg or arm by binding the injured leg to the healthy leg or the broken arm to the chest (see pg. 176 for more details on making a splint).
- Treat for shock.

GENERAL PROCEDURE—Compound Fracture

Because compound fractures include a broken bone *and* an open wound, it is necessary to treat both the break and the wound.

- Stop the bleeding by applying pressure to the wound, if possible, or to a pressure point. Use a sterile dressing, a clean cloth, or your clean bare hand (see Bleeding External pg. 7).
- Prevent infection. Let only a sterile dressing or clean hands touch the wound. Apply dressings to avoid infection, but do not apply them so tightly that they increase pain or restrict normal blood flow.
- Applying ice packs may reduce pain and swelling.
- Only medical personnel should move the victim or the broken bones.
- Do not attempt to push back a protruding bone.
- When bleeding and the threat of infection are under control, treat the injury as you would a simple fracture.

GENERAL PROCEDURE—Dislocations

Because a bone has moved out of its joint, you will note deformity, swelling, tenderness, and bruising around the affected area. Fingers, thumbs, and shoulders are most frequent sites for dislocations, but any joint may be dislocated.

- Do not try to push the bone back into place. That will increase the pain and injury.
- Treat the break as a simple fracture, keeping the affected area immobile.
- Applying an ice bag to the joint may reduce pain and swelling.

BURNS

Burns Are Classified According to Their Severity and Depth

Minor Burns

First-degree burns (e.g., sunburn)
- reddening of the skin
- no blisters
- no swelling

In first-degree burns the skin is merely reddened, as in mild sunburn. There are *no blisters,* nor is there deep tissue destruction. Another characteristic of a minor burn is that it covers a small area. If it is minor in damage but extends over much of the body, its effect may be serious.

GENERAL PROCEDURE

- Immediately apply ice or cold-water compresses. Continue this application for 30 minutes.
- Then you may apply a sterile dressing to the affected area.
- Or apply Vaseline or preparations (Solarcaine, etc.) readily available at stores.

Major Burns

Second-degree burns (partial penetration of skin thickness)
- blisters
- swelling

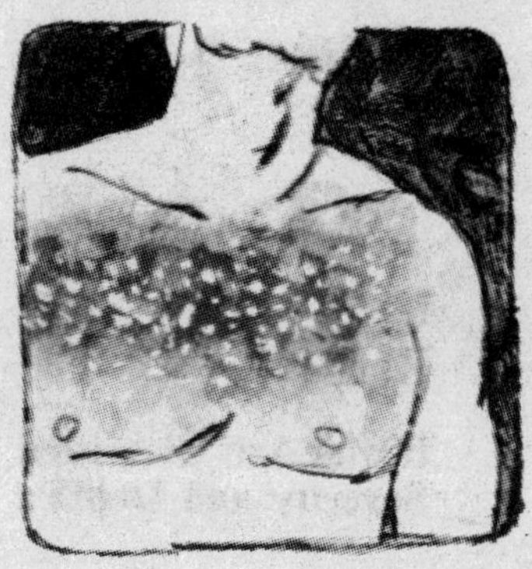
Second degree burn.

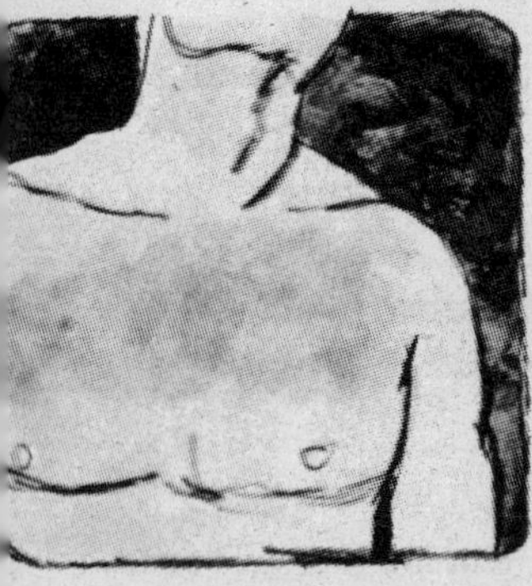
First degree burn.

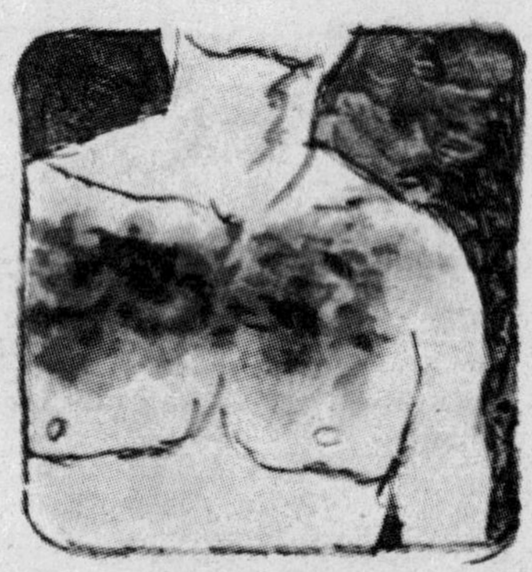
Third degree burn.

Third-degree burns (full penetration of skin thickness and may extend into fat muscle and bone)

- white or charred appearance
- there is no feeling in affected area

NOTE: The great majority of burns result from fire or other heat and are called *thermal* burns. Also common are *chemical* burns, electrical burns, and burns of the eye. (All are discussed below.) For General Procedure for second and third degree burns, see specific type of burn (i.e., chemical, thermal, etc.)

BURNS
(Chemical)

All chemical burns should be considered major emergencies. Drain cleaner, toilet cleaner, bleach, and other chemicals can burn a person's skin. Respond swiftly.

WHAT TO DO

1. Flood the burn with cold water using a hose or shower.
2. Remove the victim's clothing and shoes.
3. In most cases, treat the wound with cold water only.
4. Prevent infection.
5. Be alert for shock.
6. Have someone contact a doctor.

Read General Procedure for details.

GENERAL PROCEDURE

- Prevent infection by washing your hands with soap and warm water.
- Wash the wound with large amounts of cold water. Place the victim in a shower or under a hose, or put the affected area under cold running tap water.
- Be careful *not* to wash the chemical onto another part of the body.
- While flooding the burn with water, strip off any clothes and shoes that have come into contact with the chemical.
- If first-aid directions for the specific chemical are available on the

chemical container, follow them. Otherwise, treat the wound with water only.

- Apply a cold, wet sterile dressing that will protect against infection and keep air out.
- Be alert for the onset of shock (see pg. 79).
- Have someone contact a doctor fast.

BURNS
(Electrical)
(Also see Electric Shock, Pg. 58)

All electrical burns should be considered *major.* Burns from electricity often look minor, even when there are severe third-degree burns. Many electrical burns are caused by home appliances with exposed working parts (toasters, electric heaters) that are touched with wet hands, electric service outlets that have metal objects inserted into them and, outside the home, fallen electric wires and lightning.

The burn itself may be less dangerous than the effects the electric shock may have on the heart.

WHAT TO DO

1. Disengage the current from the victim.
2. If necessary, give CPR (see pg. 29).
3. Have someone contact a hospital ambulance.
4. Treat for shock.
5. Prevent infection.

Read General Procedure for details.

GENERAL PROCEDURE

- If the victim remains connected to an electric current, do *not* touch him. Shut off the current. Or remove the victim from the current by pushing him away from it with a nonconductor (e.g., a wooden broom handle) or pull him away with a rope. Or use a long piece of wood to remove the electric wire from contact with the victim (see pg. 58 for more details).

- *Only* after the victim is separated from the current should you touch him.
- Check his breathing. Administer CPR if necessary (see pg. 29).
- Have some one get medical help while you remain with the victim.
- Continue CPR, if necessary, until medical help arrives or you are exhausted. Although the victim may appear lifeless, he may revive after extensive attempts at resuscitation.
- Be alert for shock (see pg. 79).
- Do *not* clean the burn or disturb any blisters.
- Cover the burn with sterile dressings, clean cloths, or plastic wrap to keep air and infection out.
- Keep the patient quiet until medical help arrives.

BURNS

(Thermal)

(Also see Heatstroke, Pg. 72.)

Major Thermal Burns

Thermal burns result from fire, scalding liquids, steam, or too much sun.

WHAT TO DO

1. Have someone call an emergency ambulance.
2. Remove clothing carefully, but not if it sticks to skin.
3. Cover victim with clean sheet if the affected area is very large.
4. Flood victim or affected area with cold water.
5. Treat the victim for shock.

Read General Procedure for details.

GENERAL PROCEDURE

- Have someone call a hospital ambulance.
- Remove clothing that comes off easily. Do *not* try to remove fabric or debris that clings to the burn—cut around it.
- Wash your hands thoroughly with soap and warm water as a precaution against infection.
- Immerse the affected area in clean, cold water for five minutes.
- Do *not* break blisters, as that will increase the chance of infection.
- Do *not* apply any ointments.

- Have the patient lie down and remain still.
- Treat for shock (see pg. 79). Death from thermal burns most often results from *shock*, not the burns. (In shock resulting from a burn, the liquid part of the blood rushes to the affected area, leaving too little blood volume to keep the other organs functioning properly.)
- Do *not* rub the injury.
- If medical help will arrive quickly, let the burn remain open to the air. Otherwise, dress the burn. The dressing should be sterile, or at least clean, and cold and wet, to prevent infection. Apply sterile gauze pads or clean sheets. Wrap the dressing smoothly, gently, and evenly. If no cloth material is available, plastic wrap or plastic bags will prevent infection from reaching the burn.
- If you must provide transportation, have the victim lie flat, on a stretcher if possible. For arm or hand burns, elevate the extremity above the level of the body. For extensive body burns and burns of the lower extremities, prop the legs up carefully.
- Give the following fluid *only* if the victim is conscious, he wants to drink, he is not vomiting, and medical help will be delayed for more than one hour.

  ½ teaspoon of baking soda
  and 1 teaspoon of salt
  dissolved in 1 quart of water.

  Every 15 minutes, give the victim *half* a glass of this solution.
- A badly burned limb should also be splinted (as if it were a fracture) to prevent motion of burned tissue.

Minor Thermal Burns

When a thermal burn is minor, you will note only reddening of the skin, as in mild sunburn or mild burns from scalding liquids or steam.

GENERAL PROCEDURE

- Wash your hands with soap and warm water to prevent infection.
- Bring the burn to cold water or bring cold water or ice to the burn.
- Keep the affected area in cold water for up to one half hour. This prevents infection from reaching the wound and cools it, which should help to reduce the pain.
- When the pain subsides, remove the burn from the cold water or remove the cold compresses from the burn.
- *Only* if there are *no* blisters, apply petroleum jelly, mineral oil, or a commercial ointment.
- Do *not* apply butter or margarine to any burn; both contain salt, which will increase the pain.
- Cover the affected area with a sterile compress, bandaged gently in place, to prevent infection.
- Contact a doctor.
- Give the adult patient one or two aspirin for pain.

26

BURNS

(Eye)

All eye burns are major emergencies. They result from thermal sources (a spark from a fire) or from chemicals.

Chemical Burns

Chemicals sometimes accidentally get into the eyes. When this happens, wash out the eye immediately.

WHAT TO DO

1. Flood the victim's eye with water.
2. Cover the eye with thick compress.
3. Seek medical attention immediately.

GENERAL PROCEDURE

- Hold open the victim's eye as you place his head under a faucet. (The worse the victim's pain the more urgent the flushing.) The best way to flush the eye is to run tap water into it for at least 10 minutes. Be sure the affected eye is *closest to the sink,* so water with the chemical will run off into the sink and not into the other eye.
- If the victim cannot keep the eye open while it is being flooded with water, hold it open for him. Separate the upper and lower eyelids to be sure that water flushes the entire eye.

- Gently cover the eye with a small, thick compress and fasten it in place with a bandage.
- Do not let the victim rub his eye.
- Seek medical attention immediately.

RULE OF THUMB: If the chemical feels "squeaky clean," it's an acid; if it feels slippery or soapy, it's an alkali. A 5-minute irrigation is fine for acid, but alkali burns need at least a 30-minute flushing to save the cornea. After flushing, patch the eye closed.

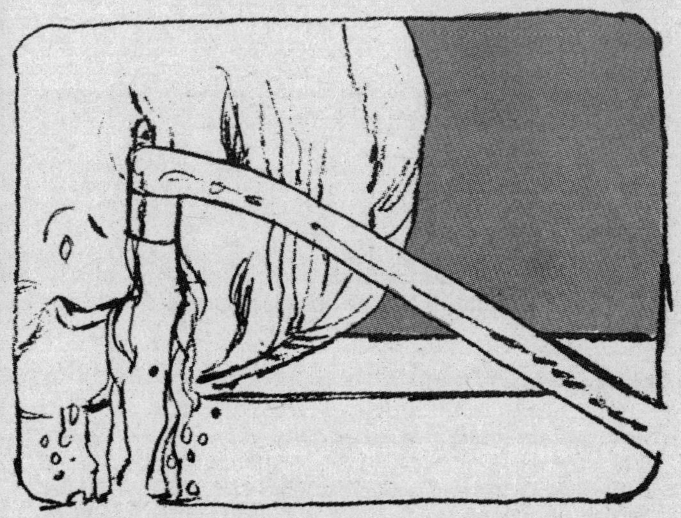

Flood eye with water.

Thermal Burns

- Follow the above procedure for flushing the eye.
- If necessary to relieve pain, place a few drops of mineral oil or olive oil into the affected eye. But put *no* other solution into an eye burned by chemicals.

CARDIOPULMONARY RESUSCITATION

(CPR)

WARNING: CPR is a combination of artificial respiration and artificial circulation. Artificial respiration (either mouth-to-mouth or mouth-to-nose resuscitation) is safe for the untrained first-aider. But artificial circulation (usually called external heart compression or external heart massage) must ONLY be applied by trained rescuers. Untrained first-aiders who attempt artificial circulation will very likely cause rib fractures, severe internal bleeding, or other complications. The American National Red Cross and the American Heart Association can direct you to excellent short courses that will teach you how to save a life using CPR.

ARTIFICIAL RESPIRATION

For human life to be sustained, the airway must be open and breathing must be maintained. Common causes of respiratory failure:

- Blocked airway
- Asphyxia
- Croup
- Drowning
- Electric shock
- Heart disease
- Strangulation
- Poisoning
- Shock.

Never give artificial respiration to a person who is breathing adequately on his own. If you are in doubt, listen, look, and touch to find out if he is breathing.

Signs and Symptoms of Respiratory Failure:
1. Blue lips, fingernail beds, and tongue.
2. Loss of consciousness.
3. Dilated pupils.
4. No visible signs of breathing.

WARNING: If the air supply is cut off, the victim will die in six minutes or less. But before you start CPR be very careful to assess the situation. If the victim is not breathing but the heart is still pumping, only apply artificial respiration, not external heart massage.

GENERAL PROCEDURE

- Have someone call a hospital ambulance.
- Place the victim on his back, with his face to the side.
- Open the victim's mouth. Quickly wipe any foreign matter from it with your fingers. You can wrap your fingers in a cloth if you like.
- Tilt the victim's head back so his chin is pointing up. *Be sure* to check the *tongue.* Respiratory failure most commonly occurs when the tongue drops back and obstructs the throat.
- To open the airway, put one hand behind the victim's neck and lift. Then place the heel of your other hand on the victim's forehead and tilt the head back as far as it will go without straining. For an infant or child lift the head so the jaw juts out.
- The tongue should be forward now. If not, pull it from the back of the throat to its natural position. Maintain the head in the backward-titled position.
- Have someone get medical help.

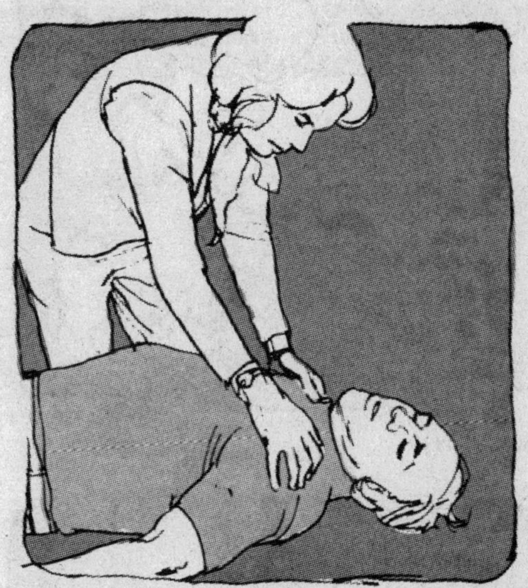

1. Place victim on his back with his face to the side.

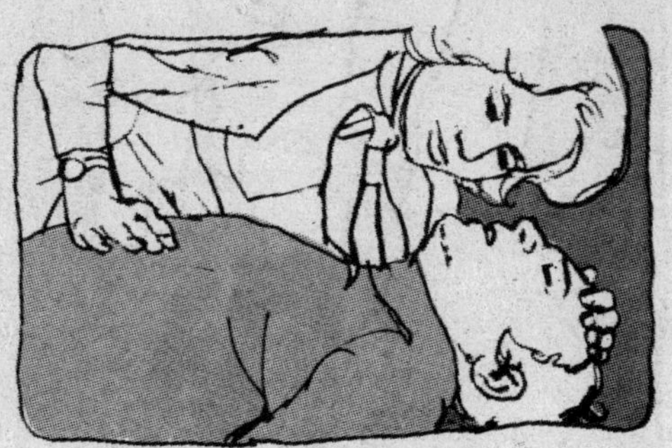

2. Check for heartbeat and/or breathing.

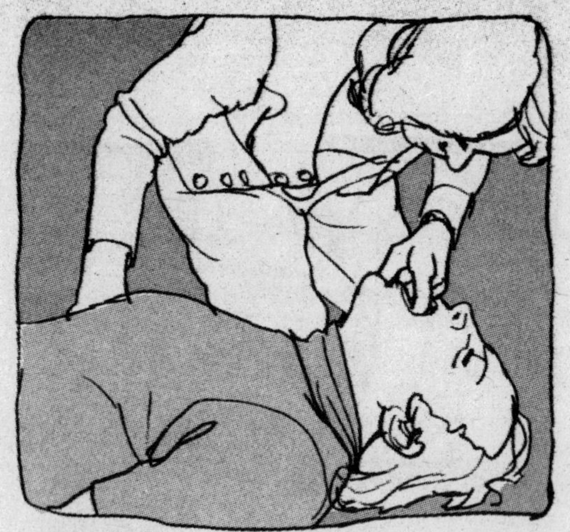

3. Clear mouth.

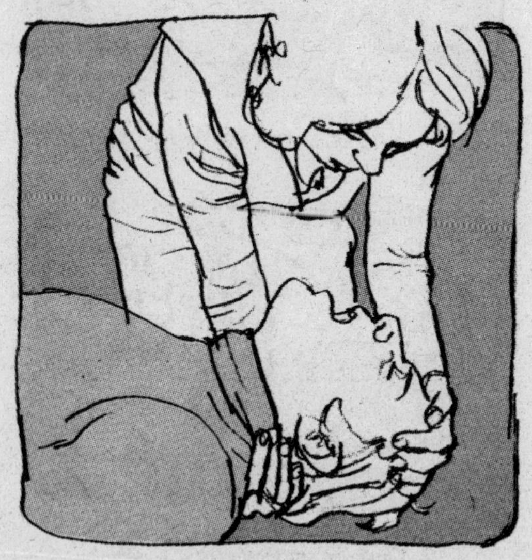

4. Tilt head back.

The most effective form of artificial respiration is the mouth-to-mouth or the mouth-to-nose method. You must actually breathe for the victim.

How to Administer Mouth-to-mouth Respiration

1. Pinch the victim's nose closed with the thumb and forefinger of the hand pressing on his forehead. Then cover his mouth with yours. If you prefer, place a handkerchief over his mouth first.

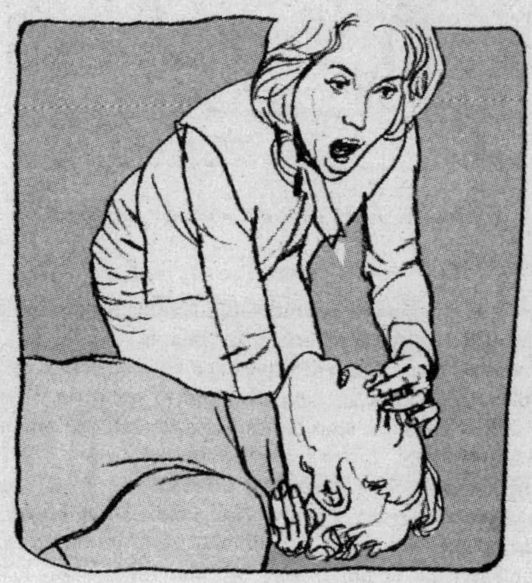

5. Pinch nose; take a deep breath.

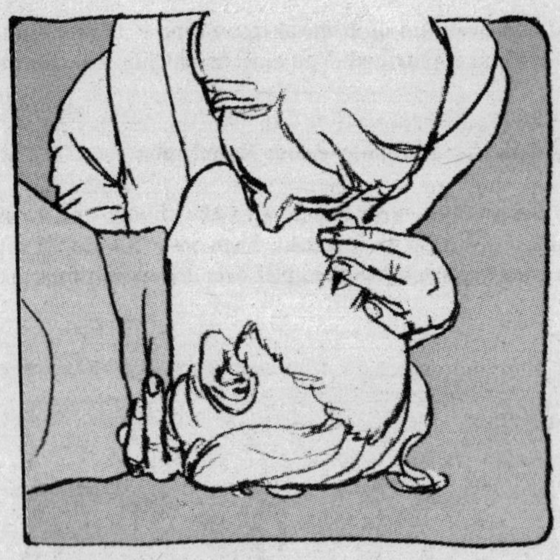

6. Blow into mouth until victim's lungs expand.

2. Now blow into the patient's mouth—full breaths for adults, shallow breaths for children, puffs of breath for infants.
3. If the airway is clear, you will experience only moderate resistance to your blowing. Watch the patient's chest to see when it rises.
4. When his chest expands, stop blowing. Raise your mouth and turn your head to the side. *Listen* for exhalation.
5. Watch the patient's chest to see that it falls.
6. Repeat—one breath every 5 seconds for adults. Small breaths every 3 seconds (about 20 breaths per minute) for children and infants.
7. Check for heartbeat or pulse every two minutes.

To Administer Mouth-to-nose Respiration

1. Maintain the patient's head in the tilt-back position with your hand on his forehead. Close his mouth with your other hand. Take a deep breath and seal your mouth around his nose. Or, for a child or infant, seal your mouth around his nose and mouth.
2. Blow into the victim's nose—full breaths for adults, shallow breaths for children, puffs of breath for infants.
3. Upon exhalation, open the patient's mouth to let air escape.

If you are not getting air exchange, recheck the position of the head and jaw. Also check the back of the mouth to see if foreign matter is obstructing air passage.

- If foreign matter is preventing ventilation, use the manual thrust as described under Choking (see pg. 41).
- *Always* continue artificial respiration until the patient breathes for himself or is pronounced dead by a doctor.

NOTE: Recovery is often rapid, except when the cause is carbon-monoxide poisoning, drug overdose, or electrical shock. In these instances it may take several hours of artificial respiration before the victim breathes on his own. Continuously check for a pulse—if there is none, administer CPR.

- Once revived, the victim of respiratory failure *must* be treated, and *must* be examined by a doctor.

ARTIFICIAL CIRCULATION

If the heart has stopped beating, the victim will shortly stop breathing too. *Always* apply artificial respiration when using artificial circulation. The possible causes of cardiac arrest are:

- blocked airway
- heart disease
- drowning
- asphyxia
- electric shock

- strangulation
- poisoning
- shock.

Never apply external cardiac massage when the heart is pumping adequately; it may result in death. Check the heartbeat by feeling each carotid pulse separately in the neck. To find the carotid pulse, first keep the victim's head tilted back, then use your index and middle fingers to locate the Adam's apple. Move your fingers laterally to the groove between the trachea and the muscles at the side of the neck, and you will feel the carotid pulse.

If there is no carotid pulse on both sides, begin CPR immediately. It is absolutely essential to be certain there is no pulse and no heartbeat *before* beginning cardiac massage.

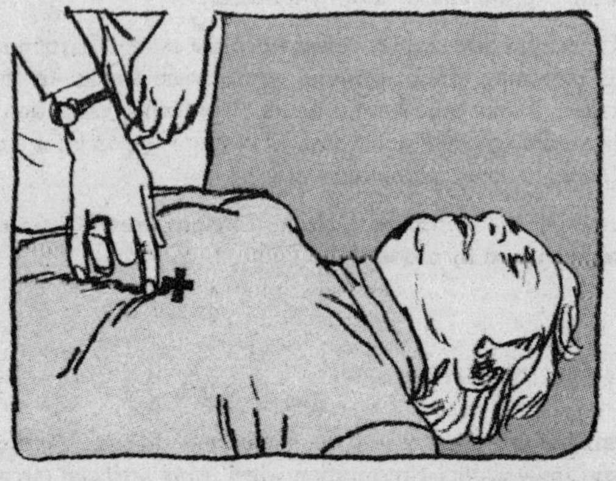

Measure up two fingertips from tip of xiphoid.

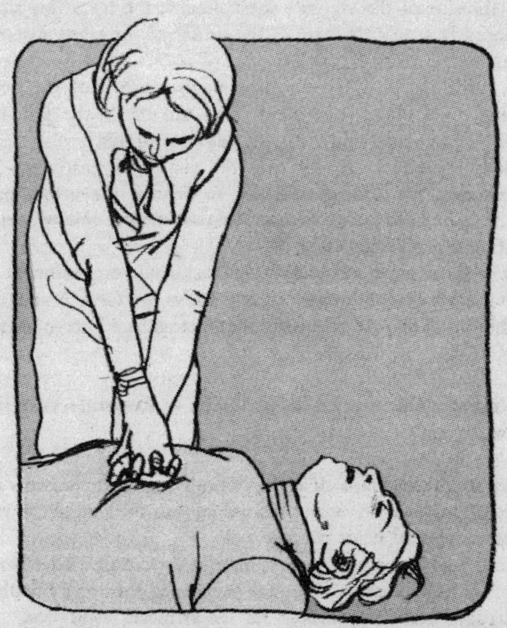

Depress victim's lower sternum 1½ to 2 inches.

GENERAL PROCEDURE

If ONE Rescuer Discovers an Adult Victim of Respiratory Failure and Cardiac Arrest

- Tilt the head back.
- Give four rapid mouth-to-mouth breaths.
- Check for carotid pulse.
- *Only if trained* in external heart compression, proceed by making sure the victim is lying on his back on a firm surface. Place yourself

close to the side of the victim's chest. Locate the tip of his xiphoid (the xiphoid is a delicate bone in the center of the chest just below the breastbone), measure up about 1 1/2 inches from the tip of the xiphoid, place the heel of your hand in the middle of the victim's breastbone, then place your other hand on top of the first hand. Interlock your fingers, and keep your elbows straight.

- Bring your shoulders directly over the victim's breastbone. Exert pressure downward almost vertically to depress the breastbone at least 1 1/2 to 2 inches (3.5 to 5 cms.). Relaxation must follow compression and be of equal duration.
- Perform both artificial circulation and artificial respiration in a 15 to 2 ratio: after every 15 chest compressions, perform 2 very quick lung inflations. The rate of chest compressions is 80 per minute.

If TWO Rescuers Discover an Adult Victim of Respiratory Failure and Cardiac Arrest

- One rescuer positions himself at the victim's head and performs artificial respiration, and the second rescuer goes to the side of the victim and applies external heart compression.
- The compression rate is 60 per minute in a ratio of 5 to 1, so that five external heart compressions are performed for every breath. Do not interrupt chest compressions for the artificial respiration.
- When the rescuers tire, they can switch positions quickly.

An INFANT Victim of Respiratory Failure and Cardiac Arrest Is Treated by One Person

- Use the tips of your index and middle fingers (not the heel of your hand) to depress the breastbone 1/2 to 3/4 of an inch. The rate of compression is 80 to 100 per minute, with quick, light puffs of breath delivered after every five compressions.

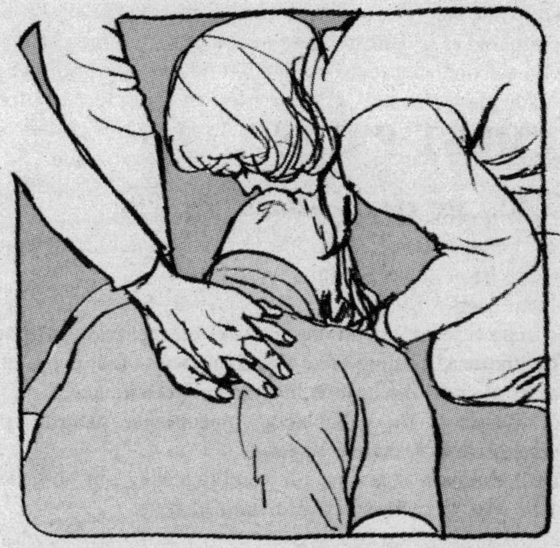

Two people working simultaneously.

To Check the Effectiveness of CPR

- Observe the victim's pupils every few minutes or as often as possible. If the pupils are dilated and do not constrict when a bright light is applied, serious brain damage has developed or is imminent. If the pupils are dilated but react to light by narrowing down, an adequate flow of oxygen and blood to the brain is indicated.
- Feel the carotid pulse after the first minute of CPR and every few minutes thereafter until the carotid pulse is sustained and breathing is spontaneous.
- Continue CPR until ambulance arrives or until victim regains spontaneous respiration and heartbeat.

CHEST PAINS

(Also see Heart Attack, Pg. 70)

Not all chest pains are major medical emergencies. Although heart attack is the most common fear associated with chest pains, other possible causes of chest discomfort include indigestion, gas, food poisoning, ulcers, diseases of the gall bladder, pneumonia, pleurisy, pulmonary emboli, and rib and muscle diseases.

Even if the pain is severe, the condition may not be serious, but it would be wise to consult a doctor immediately.

WHAT TO DO

1. Have someone call a hospital ambulance.
2. Give no food or drink.
3. Reassure patient.
4. Be prepared to transport patient.

Read General Procedure for details.

GENERAL PROCEDURE

- Give nothing by mouth—*no* laxatives, *no* water, and *no* alcoholic beverages, any of which could increase the pain and cause vomiting.
- Contact a doctor to get advice.
- Place the patient in the position of greatest comfort.
- It is best to have the patient transported by trained medical personnel if possible, but be prepared to rush the patient to a hospital yourself. If possible, have him lie down while being transported.
- Be as calm and reassuring as possible. Any anxiety or worry you show will increase the patient's fears.

CHOKING

Choking *always* has the potential to be a major medical emergency. Without air, the brain can survive undamanged for only about four minutes.

Signs and Symptoms of Choking

1. The victim cannot talk.
2. He signals distress by grabbing his neck.
3. He has difficulty inhaling.
4. He makes choking sounds.
5. His lips, tongue, or fingernails are bluish.

How to Recognize Choking When the Victim Is Unconscious

1. Listen for breathing.
2. Check the throat for blockage.
3. Begin artificial respiration.
4. If the victim's chest does not rise with each breath, the air passage is blocked.

CAUTION: The *only* completely safe way to remove a foreign body obstructing an airway is for the victim to cough up and expel the object. Giving blows to the back may cause the object to travel farther down the windpipe. Administering manual thrusts may cause internal injuries. And using your fingers to remove the object may, instead, push the object farther into the throat. Special training, most often in conjunction with Cardiopulmonary Resuscitation (CPR), is available from the American National Red Cross and through the American Heart Association.

NOTE: There are two widely recognized procedures that can be applied to choking victims: the Heimlich Maneuver and the Red Cross technique of back blows and manual thrusts.

Dr. Henry J. Heimlich, a Cincinnati surgeon, developed the Heimlich Maneuver, which is also called the "Hug of Life" "abdominal thrusts" and the "manual thrust." To use his technique, the rescuer stands behind or kneels astride the victim and uses one hand to press the other sharply upward into the victim's abdomen, just below the rib cage. This manual thrust causes a rush of air through the windpipe, forcing the foreign matter out.

The American Red Cross technique incorporates the use of manual thrusts in concert with a series of back blows.

Although the Red Cross technique has been widely taught, some doctors, including Dr. Heimlich, believe that back blows are not only unnecessary, but are potentially dangerous in that the foreign matter can be forced to go farther into the windpipe and valuable time is wasted.

To be as accurate and as fair as possible in this book, we feel it necessary to explain the two schools of thought on first aid for choking victims.

GENERAL PROCEDURE

If the ADULT Victim Is CONSCIOUS

- Do not confuse heart attack with choking. Ask the victim, "Can you speak? "If not, he's choking. If he can, choking is not the problem.
- Try to get him to cough up and expel the object.. He is likely to panic as soon as he realizes he can't breathe, so tell him calmly to *relax and cough.*
- Have someone call an emergency ambulance.

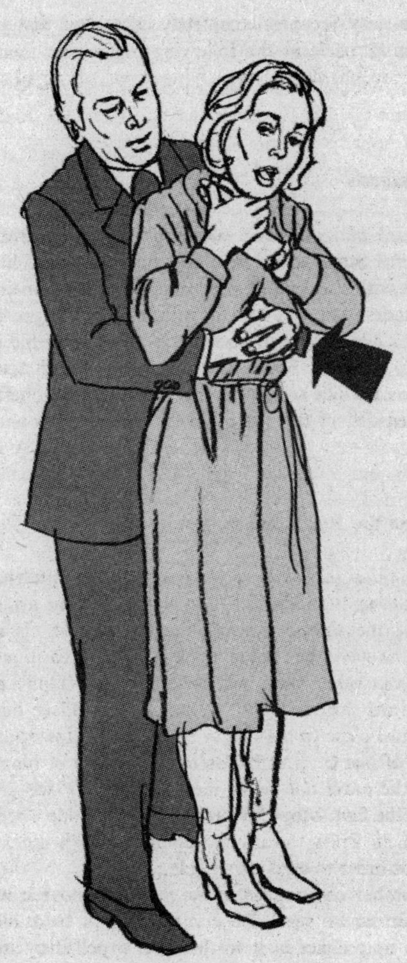

Placement of hands-standing.

- If the victim's airway becomes completely obstructed and you have the *proper training,* perform the following maneuvers immediately and in quick succession, whether he is lying down, sitting, or standing.

The Red Cross suggests

- *Perform four back blows in rapid succession.* For the victim who is *standing or sitting:* Stand at the side and slightly behind him. Give him *back blows* with the heel of your hand over his spine, between his shoulder blades. Support him by placing your other hand on his chest. If possible, his head should be lower than his chest so that gravity can be used. If the victim is *lying:* Kneel down, then roll the victim on his side so that he faces you with his chest against your knees. Then deliver the sharp blows described just above.

Both Heimlich and the Red Cross suggest

- *Perform four manual thrusts in rapid succession.* For the victim who is *standing or sitting:* Stand behind him and wrap your arms around his waist. Place the *thumb side* of your fist against his abdomen slightly above the navel but below the tip of the breastbone. Grasp your fist with your other hand and press into the victim's abdomen with quick upward thrusts. If the victim is *lying:* Place him on his back. Either kneel close to his side or straddle his hips or one thigh. Place the heel of one of your hands in the middle of his abdomen slightly above the navel but below the breastbone. Place your other hand on top of the first. Move forward so your shoulders are directly over his abdomen. Press toward the diaphram with quick upward thrusts. (Do not press toward either side.)
- *If the foreign matter can be seen in the mouth,* remove it with your fingers. If it cannot be seen, the combination of back blows and manual thrusts may dislodge it so that it is expelled by the victim or removable with your fingers.
- Have the victim examined by a doctor.

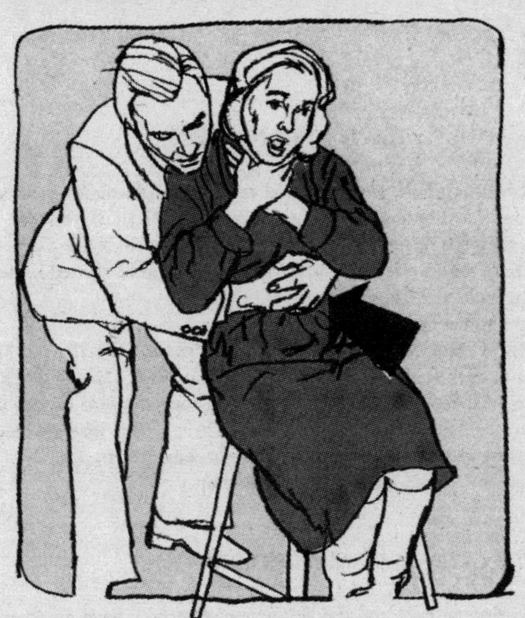

Placement of hands-sitting.

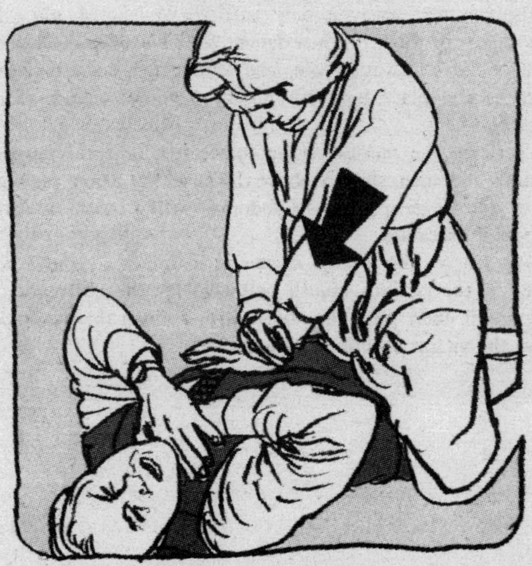

Placement of hands-lying.

If the ADULT Victim Is UNCONSCIOUS

- If breathing fails, start artificial respiration (discussed in this section under Cardiopulmonary Resuscitation [CPR]). If you can breathe for the victim, his airway is not completely blocked.
- If there is no pulse, cardiac massage must also be started if the patient is to have any hope of survival.
- Have someone get medical help.
- If the victim cannot breathe and you cannot breathe for him, and you have the *proper training,* perform four *back blows* in quick succession (discussed above). Then perform four *manual thrusts* in quick succession (discussed just above). Then, if the foreign matter can be seen in his mouth, remove it with your fingers.
- Have the victim examined by a doctor.

For INFANTS and SMALL CHILDREN

It is safest to perform the following after you have received *proper training.*

- If the victim's airway is only *partially* obstructed, place him face down on your forearm, then deliver *back blows* (as discussed above).
- If the victim's airway is *completely* obstructed, angle his head downward as you place him face down on your forearm, then deliver *back blows.*
- To perform the *manual thrust,* place two or three fingers on the victim's abdomen, slightly above the navel but below the breastbone. Press your fingertips into his abdomen with a quick, upward thrust. Repeat if necessary.
- If you can see the foreign matter in his mouth, remove it. Do *not* probe in the victim's mouth or throat for the obstruction, as this action will likely push the object farther down the windpipe.
- Have the victim examined by a doctor.

CONVULSIONS AND EPILEPSY

Convulsions (also called seizures) are attacks of unconsciousness, usually accompanied by violent muscular contractions at the beginning, that can be caused by an acute infectious disease, high fever, a head injury with brain damage, a brain tumor, or epilepsy.

Epilepsy is a chronic disease, usually with no known cause, that is characterized by repeated convulsions.

The signs and symptoms of convulsions and epilepsy include loss of consciousness, and often the eyes will roll, there will be frothing at the mouth, clenched teeth, and the muscles will twitch and jerk. If the victim is standing when the attack occurs, he will fall.

WHAT TO DO

1. Have someone call a hospital ambulance.
2. Get victim onto the floor.
3. Remove objects from the victim's vicinity.
4. Never try to stop convulsions.
5. Watch the victim's breathing.
6. Contact your doctor.

Read General Procedure for details.

GENERAL PROCEDURE

- If the victim tells you an attack is imminent, ease him onto the floor on his back.
- Loosen tight clothing.

- Push away any nearby objects. The greatest threat to the victim is from *injuries* as a result of contact with dangerous objects (tables, chairs, lamps, glass, etc.).
- *Never* try to stop convulsions. Let them run their course, no matter how frightening they appear.
- Try to place a folded handkerchief between the victim's teeth, to keep him from biting his tongue and lips.
- Keep the victim lying down.
- *Make sure* his airway is open.
- To prevent his inhaling vomit into his lungs, turn the victim's head to the side or have him lie on his stomach.
- Note that breathing may stop near or at the end of the convulsions. But breathing usually resumes spontaneously. If it does not resume, give artificial respiration (see pg. 29).
- After the convulsions are over, let the victim sleep or rest. He will remain unconscious for 5–30 minutes and is usually incoherent when first awakened.
- Contact your doctor for advice on future actions.

CROUP

Croup is a form of laryngitis in infants and young children.

Signs and Symptoms of Croup:
- Hoarseness.
- Barking cough.
- Difficult breathing.
- Fever may or may not be present.

CAUTION: Call a doctor promptly. Croup is a serious illness.

WHAT TO DO

1. Have the victim breathe steam.
2. Contact a doctor immediately.

Read General Procedure for details.

GENERAL PROCEDURE

- Prompt relief should result from filling the bathroom with steam from the shower and placing the victim in the room.
- Before returning the victim to his bedroom, provide steam in that room too, and dress him in dry sleepwear.
- Contact a doctor for advice and help.

DIABETIC COMA

(Also see Insulin Shock, pg. 74.)

Diabetic coma results when a diabetic does not take insulin on schedule, eats improperly and does not take enough insulin, or contracts an infection or other illness.

Signs and Symptoms of Diabetic Coma:

- Key sign is sickly-sweet breath (odor of nail-polish remover).
- Flushed face.
- Cherry-red lips.
- Dry skin.
- Patient appears to have a fever, but his temperature is normal or low.
- Breathing may be rapid.
- The patient may become confused and disoriented.

Sometimes, his actions and his breath odor may cause people to think he's drunk, when he needs medical attention fast. Look for a bracelet or pendant identifying him as a diabetic.

GENERAL PROCEDURE

- Have someone call an emergency ambulance. The victim requires hospitalization.
- Treat the patient for shock (see pg. 79).
- If the victim is conscious, give him sugar. If your diagnosis of diabetic coma is wrong and it is insulin shock (see pg. 74), you may save his life. If your diagnosis is correct, sugar will not hurt him.
- It may be best to place the patient in a semireclining position. Whatever position is most comfortable for him, however, be prepared for vomiting by turning his head to one side so that the vomitus cannot be inhaled into his lungs.

51

DROWNING

IMPORTANT: Drowning people will grab their rescuer, endangering their own and their rescuer's lives. So unless you are trained in life saving, do *not* attempt rescue by swimming. And because most drownings occur within reach of safety, swimming rescues usually are not necessary.

GENERAL PROCEDURE

- Call for help.
- If the victim is near the side of a pool or a dock, lie down and extend your hand or foot.
- If the victim is out of reach, extend a belt, towel, oar, rope, pole, or life preserver. Even a submerged person will grab instinctively at an object that touches him.
- If the victim is farther from safety, wade into waist-deep water with an object to extend such as a board.
- If the victim is far from safety and a rowboat is available, get it to him *stern* (back of the boat) first—stem first might cause the craft to capsize. Or extend an oar and bring the victim to the stern, where he can hang on while you row to safety.
- If the victim is unable to hold onto an oar or the stern, check him for injuries and, carefully, pull him aboard.
- Drowning victims usually die from *lack of air,* not water in the lungs or stomach. So do not try to get water out of him. Artificial respiration as well as artificial circulation should begin immediately if there is no pulse (see CPR, pg. 29).
- Have someone get medical help.
- Keep victim warm (not hot) and be alert for shock (see pg. 79).

NOTE: The victim will need medical attention—even if he appears to have recovered fully. Drowning victims often develop pneumonia and a variety of other complications from a few hours to a day or two later. Also note: Where diving boards are present, the drowning victim may have a head injury (due to striking the board or bottom of pool) or possibly a broken neck.

ICE RESCUE

NOTE: In all cases, it is safest to tie a strong rope around the rescuer's waist. Leave the free end in the hands of people who are staying a safe distance from the victim.

GENERAL PROCEDURE

- Make every effort to calm the victim. Thrashing around will cause the ice to crack further.
- The best rescue device is a ladder. Even if the ice breaks under the

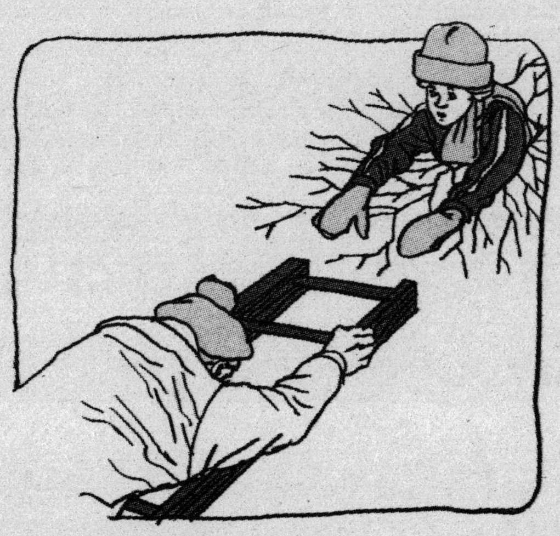

victim and rescuer, the ladder will angle upward out of the broken-ice area and support their weight. Slide the ladder out to victim so he can grasp its end.

- If you can't get near the victim, attach a strong rope to a ring buoy (or to a weight such as a hockey stick), and slide it along the ice to the victim. Provide a loop on the weighted end. Make the loop big enough for him to place his head and one arm through.
- If you must get to the victim and you have access to planks or boards, use two of them. Spread your weight as widely as possible as you lie on one board, shove the other ahead, move onto it, then bring the other ahead. Have the victim grab one of the boards, if possible.
- If the rescuer must grab the victim, the rescuer should wear skates, which he can dig into the ice to prevent being pulled into the water by the victim.
- Once the victim is out of the water, get him indoors, change him into dry clothing, and treat him for exposure or hypothermia (see Exposure, pg. 193).

DRUG OVERDOSE

(Also see Drug Abuse, pg. 121.)

It is sometimes difficult to distinguish among various types of drugs by simply observing the victim. Try to identify the substance(s) by discovering pills, capsules, other drug containers, needle marks on the victim's body, or drug-related items such as hypodermic needles, vials, eye-droppers, teaspoons, cigarette papers, or collapsible tubes. One sign is pinpoint pupils, and there may be "tracks" on arms, legs, or other areas of the body.

The following treatment can be an effective reaction to most incidents of abuse of alcohol, depressants, hallucinogens, inhalants, narcotics, stimulants, and tranquilizers.

WHAT TO DO

1. Artificial respiration may be necessary.
2. Have someone contact a doctor.
3. Be sure the airway is open.
4. Reassure the victim.
5. Beware of unpredictable behavior.

Read General Procedure for details.

GENERAL PROCEDURE

- If breathing stops, give artificial respiration (see pg. 29).
- In any critical case, stay with the victim and have a third party contact medical personnel.

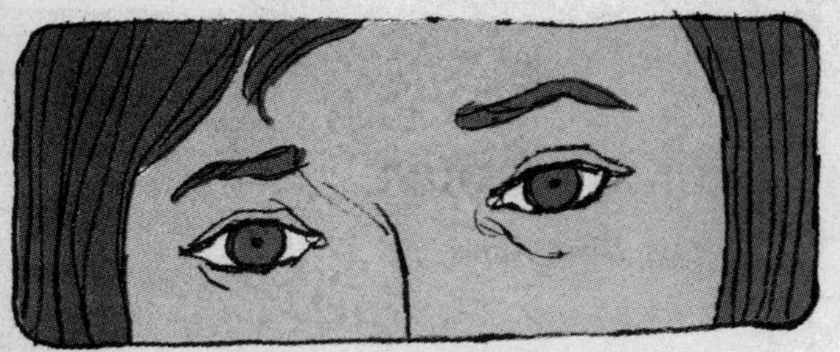

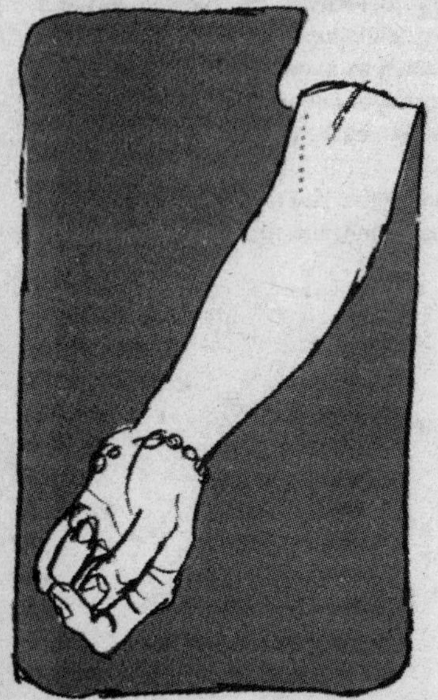

Victim may have pinpoint pupils and "tracks" on arms or other area of body.

- Make sure that neither foreign objects, vomitus, nor the tongue blocks the victim's air passage.
- Maintain his body temperature by covering him, if necessary.
- If hallucinogens are suspected (including LSD, mescaline, and other substances that cause good or bad "trips"), be aware that the victim might hurt himself and/or others. Reassure him, to help counteract nightmarish impressions. Try to maintain a constant gentle conversation.
- If depressants, inhalants, or stimulants are suspected or the victim is having delusions or hallucinations or becomes unconscious, you will have to rely on professional help.
- Be sure to give any evidence of drug abuse to the trained personnel.
- If only alcohol is suspected and the patient's color, breathing, and pulse are normal, let him sleep it off. Check the patient frequently. But if signs of shock appear (such as cold and clammy skin, rapid pulse, and abnormal breathing), get medical help (see Shock pg. 79). Be aware that an intoxicated person can harm himself and/or others. (See pg. 121 for more information on drug abuse.)

ELECTRIC SHOCK

(Also see Burns [Electrical], pg. 21.)

React as fast as possible to break the contact between the victim and the electric current. Otherwise respiratory failure or cardiac arrest may occur.

Be careful you don't become a second victim by touching the patient or the source of electricity with your bare hands or any conductive object.

WHAT TO DO

1. Disengage current from victim
2. Be prepared to give CPR (see pg. 29.)
3. Have someone contact an emergency ambulance.
4. Treat for shock.

Read General Procedure for details.

GENERAL PROCEDURE

- Shut off the electric current immediately. Disconnect the plug or pull the main switch at the fuse box.
- If that's not possible, remove the victim from contact with the current, but be very careful. Do *not* make contact with him, or you will be exposed to the same degree of shock. Stand on a dry board or on dry, nonconducting material (rubber-soled shoes or rubbers). Cover your hand with thick, nonconducting material (rubber, several layers of dry cloth) and pull him.

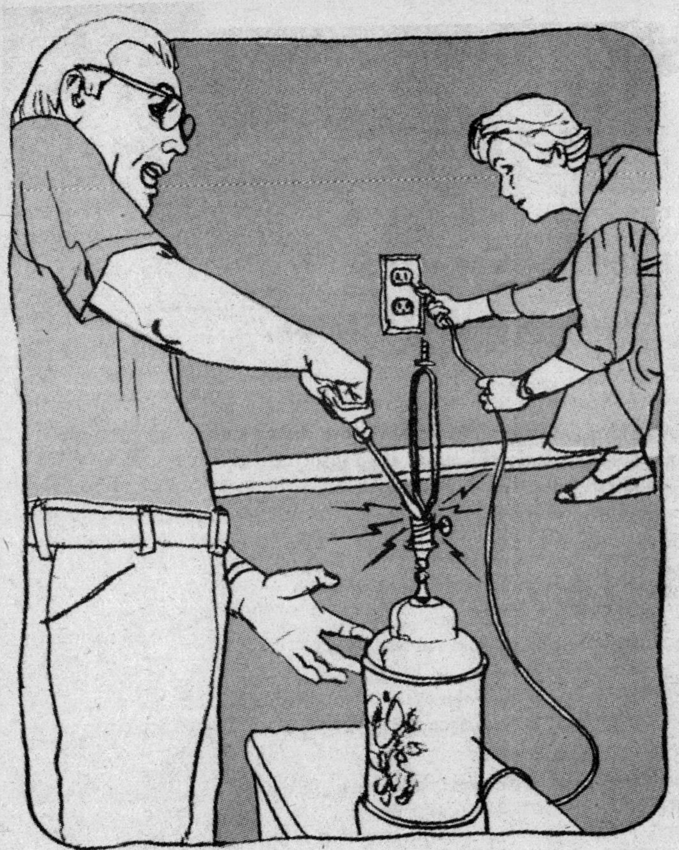

- Another rescue method is to use a dry stick or dry rope to remove the wire from the victim or the victim from the wire. Be sure your hands are dry and you are standing on a dry surface (if not, stand on a dry board). Make a loop of the rope on the stick, then place the rope over the victim's foot or hand, pulling him to safety. This method might also be used to pull the wire away from the victim.
- If necessary, start cardiopulmonary resuscitation (see pg. 29). Continue it until medical help arrives.
- Have someone contact a hospital ambulance.
- Treat the victim for shock (see pg. 79).

EYE INJURIES

(Also see Eye in the Index)

All but the slightest injuries to the eye should receive prompt medical attention. Foreign objects in the eye or on the inner surface of the eyelid can cause serious damage if they scratch the surface or become embedded in the eye.

WHAT TO DO

1. Keep the victim from rubbing his eye.
2. Make the eye tear.
3. Use water to wash the eye.
4. Check the inner surface of the eyelid.
5. Contact a doctor.

Read General Procedure for details.

GENERAL PROCEDURE

When foreign matter is in the eye:

- Keep the victim from rubbing his eye.
- Have the victim blink his eye many times, in hopes that tears will wash away the offending object.
- If the object remains and you want to examine the eye, wash your hands first with soap and warm water.
- Bring the victim's upper eyelid down over the lower for a moment, with the eye turned up. Tears will flow, perhaps washing the object out of the eye.

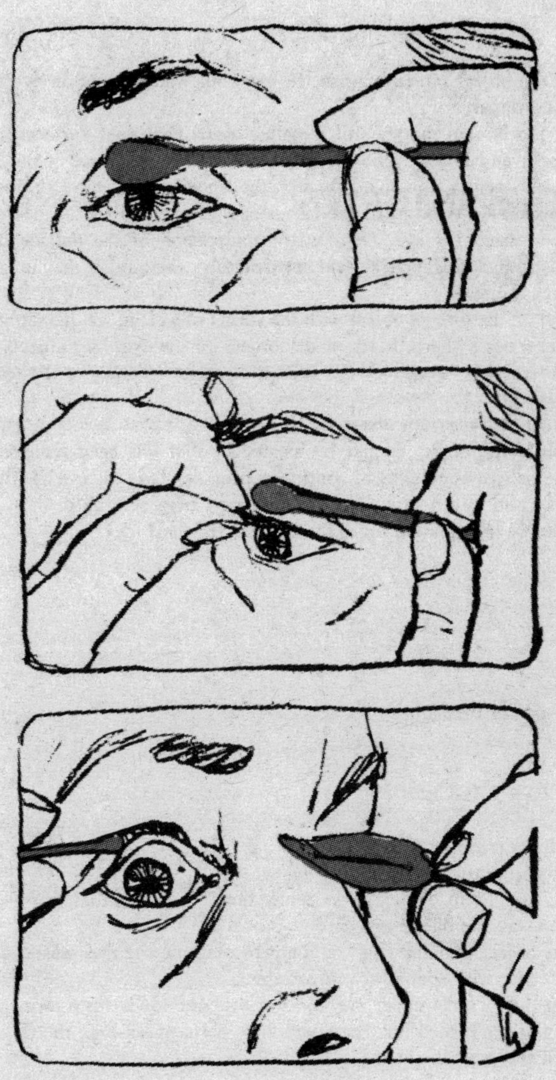

- If the object remains, wash the eye with water, using an eyecup or eyedropper.
- If the foreign matter still remains, check the inner surfaces of the upper and lower eyelids. To examine the inner surface of the lower eyelid, gently pull it down. For the upper eyelid, have the patient look down, then grasp the lashes and gently pull the lid down and away from the eye. Depress the midportion of the outside of the lid with a matchstick held horizontally, then raise the lid gently over the stick.
- Lift off the foreign object with the corner of a clean wet handkerchief. *Never* use a sharp, hard, or dry object on the eye. Dry objects stick and remove layers of cells (like a cigarette sticking to the lip and tearing).
- Flush the eye with water.
- But if the object cannot be located or if it has been removed yet the patient complains of continued pain, bandage the eye lightly and take him to a doctor. The eye may have been scratched.

For more information on eye problems, see the Index.

63

FAINTING

Fainting results when the brain receives a reduced supply of blood for a short time. Most often, the victim recovers consciousness when he falls or is placed in a reclining position.

The most serious aspect of fainting usually is the injury that occurs in the fall.

It is possible, however, that fainting is a sign of an important underlying illness.

WHAT TO DO

1. Ease the victim onto the floor.
2. Check his breathing.
3. Never throw water on the victim's face.
4. Determine if there are injuries from the fall.
5. If the victim remains unconscious, contact a doctor.

Read General Procedure for details.

GENERAL PROCEDURE

- If a person feels faint, ease him into a reclining position or bend him over with his head at knee level.
- If the victim has fallen down, leave him lying down.
- Loosen tight clothing.
- Try to keep people away.
- Make sure the victim is breathing well. If necessary, check the tongue to make sure it is forward. You may have to pull it forward with your fingers.

- If the victim vomits, roll him on his side or turn his head to the side so the vomitus does not cause choking.
- *Never* throw water on the victim's face, because of the danger of aspirating the water into the lungs. You can, however, gently bathe the face with cool water.
- Be sure the victim is completely revived before giving him any liquids.
- If you like, you may wave smelling salts or ammonia under his nose.
- Determine if the victim's fall has caused any injuries.
- If recovery is prompt, there may be no need to contact a doctor. But if the victim is unconscious for several minutes, have somone seek medical assistance.

FALLS

Among the many injuries caused by falls are internal and external bleeding; bone fractures; head, neck, and pelvis injuries; and unconsciousness (see these subjects in this section).

WHAT TO DO

1. Keep the victim still.
2. Check his breathing.
3. Stop any bleeding.
4. If the victim is unconscious, have someone get medical help.
5. Be alert for shock.

Real General Procedure for details.

GENERAL PROCEDURE

- Do *not* move the victim (unless his present position is dangerous). Movement may cause further damage and pain.
- Make sure the victim can breathe easily. If not, be prepared to give him artificial respiration (see pg. 29).
- Stop any major bleeding (see pg. 7).
- If the victim is unconscious, have someone get medical help.
- If the victim is conscious, ask what pains he feels. Provide reassurance.
- If injuries are extensive, be prepared to treat for shock (see pg. 79).
- It is always safest to have the patient examined by a physician.

FEVER

(Also see Fever [Slight] pg. 132.)

Fever is a symptom of illness. It is one of the body's ways of fighting off infection. Although it produces discomfort, fever itself is seldom harmful, except when it reaches high levels.

For infants and young children, a fever of over 103° F. can result in convulsions. For adults, a fever of 105° F. and above can be hazardous.

NOTE: Normal body temperature is 98.6° F.

WHAT TO DO

1. Keep a record of the victim's temperature and pulse.
2. Give him aspirin or Tylenol.
3. Give the victim lukewarm water sponge baths.
4. Contact a doctor if necessary.

Read General Procedure for details.

GENERAL PROCEDURE—Adults

- When the victim's temperature is 101° F. or above, record it and the pulse. Record the temperature every half hour until it has been reduced to normal.
- Give aspirin or an aspirin substitute to reduce the fever (see the container label for the dosage).

A sponge bath with lukewarm water can bring down the temperature. Do not use alcohol because inhalation of the vapor can cause a toxic effect.

Contact a doctor if high fever persists or is accompanied by other symptoms of illness, such as nausea, sore throat, pain, swelling, or rash.

ENERAL PROCEDURE—Infants

When the temperature is 101° F. or above, record it and the pulse. Record the temperature every half hour until it has been reduced to normal.

Give aspirin or an aspirin substitute to reduce the fever (see the container label for the dosage).

Administer a bed bath, using a washcloth and lukewarm (not cold or cool) water. Do *not* use alcohol, because the inhaled vapor may have a harmful effect. Bathe the face first, then one arm, then the other, then the neck, etc.

Contact a doctor.

HEAD INJURIES

(For more information, see the Index.)

All head injuries should be taken seriously. Unconsciousness for *any* length of time is an indication of a potentially serious injury. Other serious symptoms include profuse bleeding, noisy breathing that indicates an obstructed air passage, clear or blood-tinged fluid draining from the nose or ears, partial or complete paralysis, speech disturbance, convulsions, pupils of eyes unequal in size, pale or flushed face, and a pulse that is slow or weak.

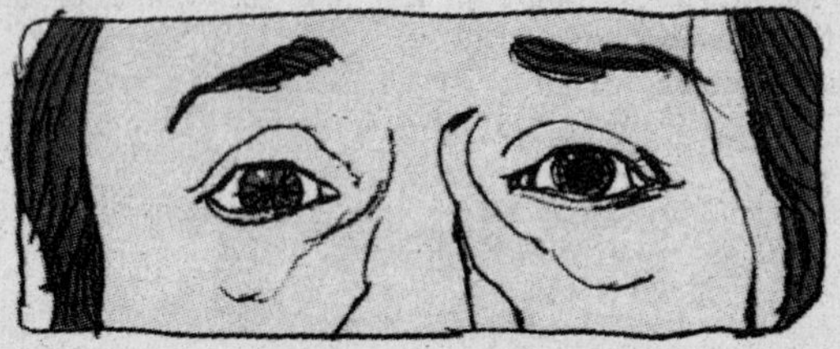

NOTE: A person with a head injury may be kept flat on his back or propped up, but the head should *not* be lower than the rest of the body, because blood will run to it.

WHAT TO DO

1. Be sure the victim is breathing properly.
2. Give him artificial respiration if needed.
3. Keep him still.
4. Have someone call a hospital ambulance.
5. Stop any bleeding.

Read General Procedure for details.

GENERAL PROCEDURE

- Make sure the victim's airway is clear. If necessary, remove any debris from his mouth and *gently* tip his head back fully, keeping his mouth closed by supporting his lower jar.
- Check for neck injuries. Often head injuries are accompanied by injuries to the neck.
- If breathing still is not proper, give artificial respiration (see pg. 29).
- If the victim is breathing well, turn his head to the side so that if he vomits, the material will drain from his mouth and not clog his lungs.
- Do *not* move the victim unless his present position endangers his life. Keep him lying down.
- If bleeding from the head injury is profuse, apply pressure to the wound (see Bleeding [External], pg. 7).
- Loosen any clothing that is tight around the neck.
- Keep the victim comfortably warm and, if necessary, treat him for shock (see pg. 79).
- Do *not* give the victim anything to eat or drink.

Minor Head Injuries

There will be no loss of consciousness, the victim's color will remain natural, and there will be no vomiting.

WHAT TO DO

1. Stop the bleeding.
2. Treat it as any wound.
3. Contact a doctor if necessary.

GENERAL PROCEDURE

- Stop the bleeding (see pg. 7) and prevent infection.
- Watch the victim closely. If he vomits, remains pale for several hours, complains of headache or dizziness after one hour, has any memory loss for events surrounding the injury, or acts drowsy or dazed, contact your doctor.

HEART ATTACK

(Also see Chest Pains, pg. 40)

Signs and Symptoms of Heart Attack

1. Anxiety—a major feature of heart attack.
2. Pain or pressure in the center of the chest, behind the breastbone, that may or may not spread down the arms or into the neck or jaw. Pain is usually described as heavy, or like a squeeze or heavy weight on chest.
3. Extreme shortness of breath.
4. Pain that is not influenced by breathing or by whether the patient sits or lies down.
5. Profuse sweating.
6. Pale and cool skin.
7. A feeling of weakness and nausea.

WHAT TO DO

1. Give the victim no food or drink.
2. Have someone call a hospital ambulance.
3. Reassure the victim.
4. Give him CPR if needed.

Read General Procedure for details.

GENERAL PROCEDURE

- Have the victim sit or lie in the most comfortable position.
- Contact medical personnel immediately. Let an expert diagnose the situation and treat it.
- If medical help cannot come to the victim, rush him to a hospital.
- Be as calm as possible. Reassure the victim, who is apt to panic and make his situation worse.
- Loosen tight clothing.
- Be prepared to give cardiopulmonary resuscitation (CPR) (see pg. 29).

HEATSTROKE

(Also see Heat Exhaustion, pg. 144, and Heat Cramps, pg. 143.)

Heatstroke (also called sunstroke) can be *fatal,* because the body cannot cool itself. Instead, the body gets hotter and hotter and the patient can no longer perspire because of dehydration.

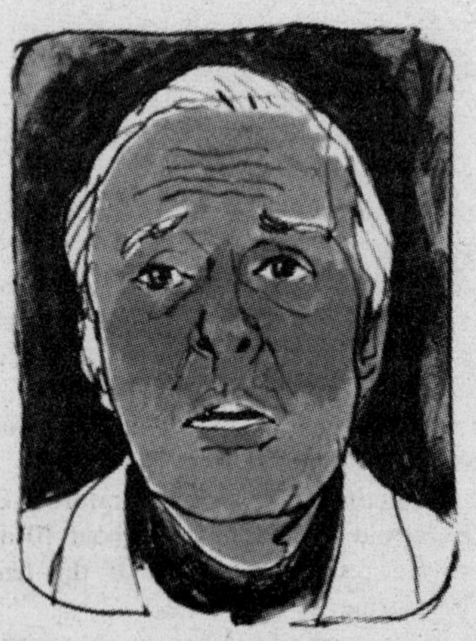

Signs and Symptoms of Heatstroke:

1. Mouth temperature is above 104° F.
2. Skin is hot, red, and dry, because the sweating mechanism isn't working.
3. Rapid, strong pulse.
4. Victim may be unconscious, irrational, or unable to move.

WHAT TO DO

1. Have someone call a hospital ambulance.
2. Cool the body.
3. Observe the victim carefully.
4. Do not overcool him.

Read General Procedure for details.

GENERAL PROCEDURE

- Immediately attempt to cool the victim's body to 102° F. Take him to the coolest place nearby. If possible, undress him, place him on his back, and spray or sponge his body with cold water. If you can't unclothe him, spray his body with cold water. Or place him in a tub of cold water, but add no ice.
- Use fans or an air conditioner, if possible, to get his temperature down to 102° F.
- A thermometer is the best means of determining his temperature. Otherwise, judge his temperature by his general condition and his pulse rate. A pulse rate below 110 beats per minute usually indicates a tolerable temperature.
- Have someone contact medical help, or take the victim to the emergency room of a nearby hospital.
- Do *not* overcool the victim. Once his temperature is down, observe him carefully. Cease cold applications for about 10 minutes. If his temperature increases, resume treatment. If the temperature decreases, provide a covering.
- *Never* give fluids to an unconscious person. A conscious victim of heatstroke can receive what he desires, except for hot fluids or stimulants.

INSULIN SHOCK

(Also see Diabetic Coma, pg. 50.)

Insulin shock results when too little sugar is in the blood, as a result of too much insulin or not enough food.

Signs and Symptoms of Insulin Shock:

1. Patient is ashen white, with moist and clammy skin covered with a cold sweat, and is in a state of shock (see pg. 79).
2. Pulse is rapid but breathing is slow and shallow.
3. There is no odor of acetone on the breath.
4. Look for a bracelet or pendant announcing his diabetic condition.

GENERAL PROCEDURE

- Because the patient lacks sugar, give it to him. If he's conscious, get it to him quickly, in the form of sugar water (2 teaspoons per glass) or orange juice. If he's semiconscious, give him small sips of sugar water or orange juice.
- If unconscious, the victim needs intravenous sugar. Do not try to put anything in mouth of unconscious person; it may get lodged in the windpipe. Call for a hospital ambulance and get the victim to a doctor or hospital immediately.

POISONING (by Inhalation)

Inhaled poisonous gases can cause death. Carbon monoxide, the most common poisonous gas, is particularly treacherous, because it has no odor.

Signs or symptoms include a victim who is unconscious and asphyxiated, with no warning other than dizziness, headache, and weakness. Death can occur in a few minutes.

WARNING: If the victim is in a closed room, garage, or other confined area, be sure to take a deep breath and hold it *before* entering.

WHAT TO DO

1. Remove the victim to clean air.
2. Have someone get medical help.
3. Keep the airway open.

Read General Procedure for details.

GENERAL PROCEDURE

- Remove the victim to fresh air.
- If that is not possible, call the fire department, police, or 911.
- Keep his airway open. If necessary, give him artificial respiration (see pg. 29).
- Loosen tight clothing.
- Do not give him alcohol of any kind.
- If you have not already done so, see that medical help is contacted. Have them bring oxygen.

POISONING (by Mouth)

(Also see Drug Abuse, pg. 121 and Drug Overdose, pg. 55.)

If someone swallows a poisonous substance, be as calm as possible while you identify the material. An uninformed or panicky reaction will make things worse. Contact a poison control center immediately for the most accurate instructions.

WHAT TO DO

1. Remove the poison from the mouth, if possible.
2. Identify the substance.
3. Have someone contact a poison control center.
4. Determine whether or not to give the victim water or to induce vomiting.
5. Be prepared to give him artificial respiration.
6. Be alert for shock.

Read General Procedure for details.

GENERAL PROCEDURE

- Remove any poison that may be in the victim's mouth.
- Identify the poison. If its container is nearby, read the label for the appropriate antidote.
- If the antidote is not immediately known, have someone contact a poison control center or medical personnel. Follow the expert advice.
- Do not give an unconscious victim water. Instead, keep him warm and get medical help immediately.

- If the victim is conscious and is not having convulsions, dilute the poison by having him drink water. Give two cups of water to children under five, a quart of water to all others. Milk is another safe liquid.
- Determine whether or not to induce vomiting. *Never* make the victim vomit if:

1. he's *unconscious* or having *convulsions*, because he could choke to death;
2. there are *burns* around the mouth, which indicate that corrosives have been swallowed and their re-entry into the throat and mouth would cause additional burns;
3. *Petroleum products* (gasoline, furniture polish, or cleaning fluids) were swallowed, because the vomitus could enter the lungs and cause pneumonia.

How to Induce Vomiting

- Tickle the back of the victim's throat with your finger.
- Give adults 1 ounce of syrup of ipecac; children, ½ ounce.

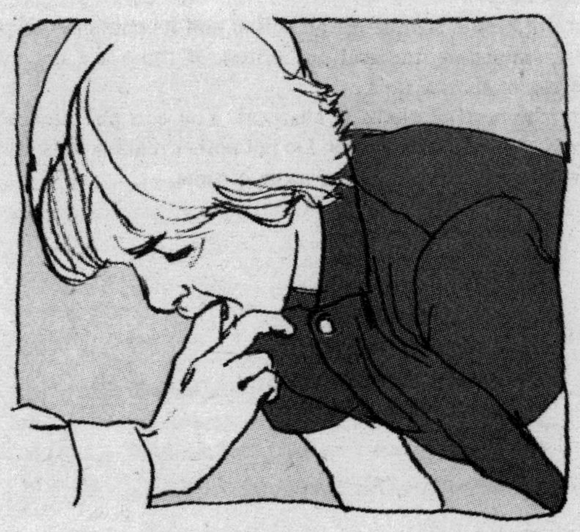

- Place the patient turned to the side, with his head lower than his hips. This prevents vomitus from entering the lungs and causing more injury. Continue to give him water and induce vomiting until the vomitus is clear.

Watch the victim's breathing. Some poisons depress respiration. If he stops breathing, give him artificial respiration (see pg. 29).

- Be prepared for shock (see pg. 79). Keep the victim warm but not hot.
- All victims of poisoning should be examined by a doctor.

Administering Antidotes

Only if you must wait for medical personnel and have done everything you can for the victim, should you prepare an *antidote* or a *demulcent.* Note that diluting the poison with water and inducing vomiting, where appropriate, are more effective remedies.

- *Demulcents* (soothing drinks) coat the lining of the stomach and intestines and help slow down the absorption of a poison. Milk, raw egg whipped in milk, or a tablespoon of olive oil in milk are the best demulcents.
- Be sure to keep a sample of the poison and its container, if possible, to be examined by medical authorities. If those are not available, save some of the vomitus.
- One of the best antidotes is charcoal. You can purchase activated charcoal at your pharmacist's. Do not bother making your own charcoal with burned toast; it is a waste of time.

79

SHOCK

Shock is a major medical emergency resulting from a depressed state of several vital body functions. During shock, the blood circulation is disturbed or even stopped due to the body's reaction to respiratory failure, profuse bleeding, poisoning, heart attack, and other serious medical conditions. The pulse is weak and rapid, blood pressure is low, and the victim is pale and clammy.

Even if the patient's injury does not prove to be critical, shock could threaten his life.

WHAT TO DO

1. Treat the injury first.
2. Keep the victim lying down, preferably on his back.
3. Keep him warm, not hot.
4. Have someone contact a hospital ambulance.
5. Raise the victim's legs about 18 inches if his injuries allow.
6. Usually, give him no fluids.
7. Loosen tight clothing.
8. Reassure him.

Read General Procedure for details.

Early Signs of Shock

1. In a light-skinned person, the skin is pale or bluish and cold to the touch. With a dark-skinned person, check for a change of color of the mucous membranes on the inside of the mouth, the underside of the eyelids, and the nail beds.
2. If the patient has perspired, the skin may be moist and clammy.

3. The victim will be weak.
4. The pulse usually will be rapid (over 100 beats per minute) but may be too faint to be felt at the wrist so feel the carotid pulse.
5. Breathing will be fast but shallow and perhaps irregular.
6. The victim probably will be nauseous.

Later Signs of Shock

1. The patient becomes apathetic and unresponsive.
2. His eyes will be sunken, with pupils dilated.
3. His skin may have a mottled appearance.

If untreated, he will lose consciousness, his body temperature will drop, and he may die.

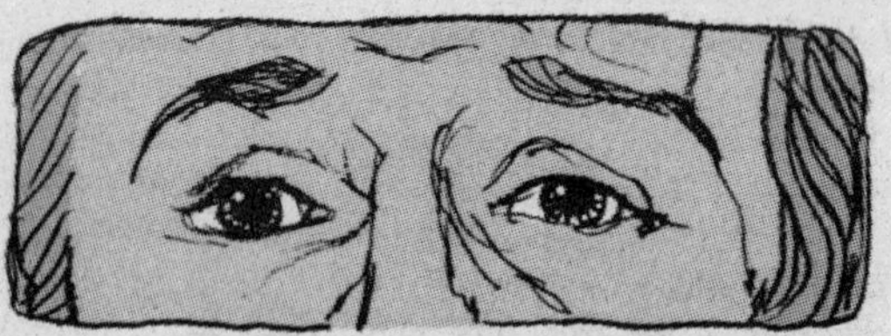

Pupils are dilated and skin is pale.

IMPORTANT: *Always treat the injury first.* For example, if the patient's breathing has stopped, give him artificial respiration. But with *every* major medical emergency, always anticipate shock and react accordingly after the injury has been controlled.

GENERAL PROCEDURE

- Keep the victim lying down, preferably flat on his back. Note that his position may depend upon the type and severity of his injury. If *neck* or *spine* injuries are possible, do not move him. If he is

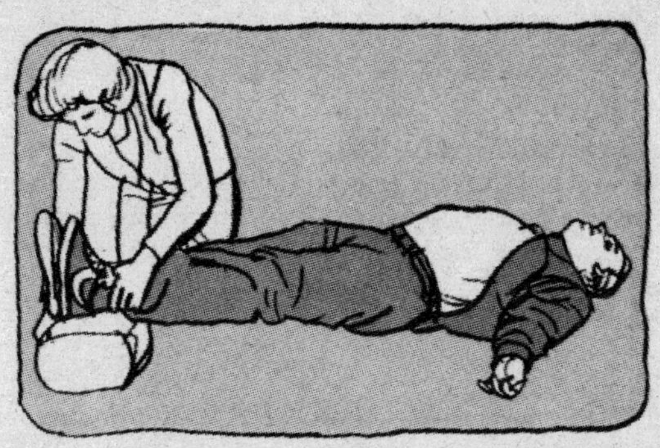

unconscious and has wounds of the *jaw* or *lower part of the face,* place him on his side, so that fluids can drain from his mouth and not block his air passage. *If in doubt* about the proper position of a shock victim, keep him *lying flat on his back.*

- If injuries do not restrict the patient's position, he may improve if his feet are raised between 12 and 18 inches. But if this causes trouble breathing or increased pain, lower the feet.
- Keep the patient warm but not hot. It may be necessary to cover him with a blanket or coat. *Be sure* he does not become too warm.
- Have someone call a hospital ambulance.
- Loosen tight clothing.
- Reassure the victim. He will probably be in pain and fearful. Tell him what you are doing for him and when professional medical help will arrive. Calm him, and you will help him greatly.
- It is safest not to give the patient any fluids. *Never* give an unconscious person anything to drink, as he might aspirate the fluid into his lungs.
- But if help will not be arriving for several hours, the patient is conscious and not having convulsions, and the cause of shock does not appear to be injury to or bleeding in the abdomen, you may give him water or a salt solution that is neither cold nor hot. The salt solution contains 1 level teaspoon of table salt and ½ teaspoon of baking soda per quart of water. Give an adult about 4 ounces (half a glass) of water or the salt solution every 15 minutes. Give half that amount to children under 12.
- *Discontinue* giving water or the salt solution if the patient becomes nauseated or vomits.

82

STROKE

A major stroke is usually caused by high blood pressure or a hardening of the arteries that results in a ruptured blood vessel in the brain or the formation of a blood clot that blocks circulation to a portion of the brain.

WHAT TO DO

1. Place the victim in a semi-reclining position.
2. Maintain breathing.
3. Have someone call a hospital ambulance.
4. Keep the victim warm.
5. Do not give him smelling salts.

Read General Procedure for details.

Signs and Symptoms of a Major Stroke

- Unconsciousness.
- Paralysis of one side of the body.
- Difficulty in breathing and swallowing.
- A mouth that is drawn to the side.
- Lack of ability to talk or a slurring of speech.
- Loss of bladder and bowel control.
- Pupils that are unequal in size.

Note, however, that there is no definite pattern of symptoms. For example, the victim of a major stroke may remain conscious or semiconscious.

GENERAL PROCEDURE

- Place the victim on his side, with his head and shoulders raised slightly.
- Maintain an open airway. If necessary, give the victim artificial respiration (see pg. 29).
- If victim has trouble breathing, place him on his side so that secretions will leave his mouth.
- Have someone get medical help immediately. If possible, obtain advice over the phone.
- Retain the victim's body heat by covering him. Do not overheat him.
- Do *not* use any stimulants such as smelling salts.

Minor Stroke

During a minor stroke, small blood vessels of the brain are blocked. The victim usually remains conscious. Other signs depend upon the location of the block and the amount of brain damage.

Watch for such signs as headache or dizziness, a sudden partial memory failure, difficulty in moving a part of the body, a speech defect, or a sudden change in disposition.

GENERAL PROCEDURE

- Protect the victim against accident or attempts at physical exertion.
- Contact medical help for advice.
- Observe the victim closely.

UNCONSCIOUSNESS

The cause of unconsciousness may be obvious. For example, a bad fall or an auto accident. Or the cause may be difficult to determine, as when the victim suffers from a heart attack, heatstroke, shock, poisoning, a stroke, or some other medical emergency.

WHAT TO DO

1. Check the victim's breathing.
2. Treat his injuries.
3. Have someone call a hospital ambulance.
4. Almost never move an unconscious person.
5. Look for emergency identification.
6. Keep the victim warm.

Read General Procedure for details.

GENERAL PROCEDURE

- Check the patient's breathing. If necessary, give him artificial respiration (see Artificial Respiration, discussed under Cardiopulmonary Resuscitation, pg. 29).
- Treat serious medical emergencies. For example, stop profuse bleeding if possible by applying pressure directly to the wound. Use a tourniquet as a last resort. (See Bleeding [External], pg. 7.)
- Have someone call a hospital ambulance immediately.
- Do *not* move an unconscious person unless his life is in jeopardy in his current position. Movement may increase his injuries and pain.
- *Never* give an unconscious person anything to eat or drink. He might choke on it or aspirate fluid into his lungs.

- Look for emergency identification around his neck, wrist, or ankle that might state the cause of his unconsciousness. If another person is present who will vouch for your actions, check the victim's wallet for information about his condition.
- Turn his head to the side, so that if he vomits, the material will drain from his mouth and not clog his lungs.
- Keep the victim warm but not hot.
- Remain with the patient until professional help arrives.
- But if you must transport the victim yourself, it is best to use a stretcher or a cot. If that is not possible, keep him lying flat and keep his body immobile.

NOTE: A faint is a temporary condition that lasts only a few moments (see Fainting, pg. 63). If a person loses consciousness for no apparent reason and does not recover in a short time, a doctor should be contacted to determine whether the victim is suffering from a simple fainting spell or a more serious condition.

SECTION TWO

Be Prepared

Anticipating medical emergencies by knowing how to react and by having the necessary supplies on hand.

The very best way to be prepared for medical emergencies is to take a first-aid course. The Red Cross, for example, offers this instruction free of charge. Some YMCAs, YWCAs, and college extension programs offer courses also. All of these choices allow you to train under experts. If you have the interest and the relatively small amount of time it takes, you'll find a first-aid training course extremely valuable.

Shorter courses are available from the same sources for people who want to learn about Cardiopulmonary Resuscitation (CPR), which is highly effective in case of a heart attack, and the Heimlich Maneuver, also called the "Hug of Life" (manual thrust or abdominal thrust), which has earned awards for preventing asphyxiation from choking. Both procedures require special training because they must be applied properly or additional injury to the patient is likely. More and more men, women, and teenagers are devoting a few hours of their free time to learn these lifesaving methods in the hopes of saving the life in an acute emergency.

This book will help you deal effectively with major medical emergencies such as severe bleeding, burns, drowning, etc. It will help you do what you can and determine what must be left to trained personnel. You will also find information on dozens of minor medical emergencies, such as flu, objects in the eye, ivy poisoning etc., as well as fire emergencies.

If and when it's possible, the best procedure is to read through an item in this book before taking any action. Then, after you understand the usual responses and the particular exceptions, act to control the situation.

But, with critical emergencies, of course, it will not be possible to read all of the information before acting. So please consider following through on these two suggestions:

First, have every adult and teenager in the family read Sections One and Two. Also have them become familiar with the remainder of the book.

And second, practice. Select two or three critical emergencies from Section One. Then have someone become the patient and treat him (do not apply CPR or the manual thrust except on rubber dummies manufactured for practice). This run-through may help you and your family avoid panic during an actual emergency.

Your attitude and emotional state during an emergency can have an influence on how valuable you are as a first-aider. If your attitude is positive and you remain calm during a stress-filled situation, the chances are you'll be a great asset to the victim. Practicing in advance will help build your self-confidence.

Although there are many types of critical medical emergencies, there are a few all-important rules for handling them.

Six Most Important Responses for Major Medical Emergencies

1. *Make sure the victim is breathing.* A clear airway must be maintained, and the individual must breathe or he will not live. If necessary, clear the airway and give artificial respiration (see pg. 29).
2. *Stop any heavy bleeding.* Because blood is essential for survival, major hemorrhaging must be stopped (see Bleeding [external], pg. 190.)
3. *Prevent further injury.* Protect the victim from further harm. Move the victim *only* if his present position puts him in jeopardy. Moving could increase external and/or internal injuries. It is usually best to have the victim lie down and remain supine until medical personnel arrive.
4. *Anticipate shock.* Major injuries are *always* accompanied by some degree of shock, in which bodily reactions slow or stop the circulatory mechanisms. Because shock can be fatal, *always* treat the victim of a major medical emergency for shock (see pg. 79).
5. *Do not do more than you know how.* Do only what is essential to save a life, *if* you know what to do. But if you have not been trained in CPR or the manual-thrust "Hug of Life," you should not attempt it.
6. *Have someone get medical help.* Whenever possible, you should treat the essential needs of the victim while someone else calls a rescue

squad, the fire department, the police, an ambulance, or a doctor.

If you haven't already done so, now is a good time to determine the various experts you would call to help in a medical emergency. Space is provided on the inside covers of the book for the appropriate names and phone numbers. Consider the following:

1. *The rescue squad,* often part of the local fire department, is usually the best-trained and fastest to respond. Check to see if these paramedics are available in your community.
2. *911,* the special emergency telephone number, will bring help fast. Some localities, however, do not yet have this service.
3. *The police* may or may not be able to respond immediately with medically trained personnel.
4. *An ambulance service* may or may not bring well-trained personnel to you fast. Before an emergency, contact the local medical society for the name of the best ambulance service where you live.
5. *The telephone operator* ("0") will get you the help you need, but the call may take longer than dialing directly.
6. *Your personal or family physician* may or may not be available and may or may not be able to respond immediately.
7. *The poison-control center,* in some communities, will give information only to doctors. Call before an emergency to see if the one where you live will assist private citizens.

Vital information to give to Medical Help Over the Phone

1. *Where is the victim?* Give the city or town, street name, and street number. If calling at night, give a brief description of the house or apartment building. Get some outside lights on.
2. *What has happened?* Tell the nature of the emergency (woman is bleeding badly, child has swallowed poison, man has fallen and is unconscious).
3. *Who is calling?* Give your name. If different from the name of the homeowner or apartment dweller, give that person's name too. If neighbors are asked for directions, they may react more quickly to the occupant's name than to the address.
4. *Your phone number.* In case they have trouble with directions, etc.

5. *Will they need extra help?* If the victim is overweight, there may be a need for extra help or if there are several flights of winding stairs, etc.
6. *Any questions?* Pause and let the person on the other end of the line ask some questions.

This information will take only a matter of seconds to relate. Speak as clearly and distinctly as possible and *remain calm.* Professional help will be on its way momentarily.

If you have children, teach them to use the information on these pages. A child of four, for example, can be taught to dial "0" or to run to a neighbor's home for help. It might be good to go through this material page by page with a youngster if he or she is mature enough to understand and be able to use it.

Children and all others that you live with should know where the home medical supplies are kept. If and when an item is used, it should be returned or replaced promptly.

FIRST-AID SUPPLIES

It's best to keep all of the first-aid supplies together, perhaps on one shelf of the medicine cabinet or, better yet, in a special container. The bathroom and the kitchen are logical places to store the container. And when you go away for trips, be sure to take the container with you—or have a second one in the car. Also, you might want to keep this book with your medical supplies.

Many pharmacies and other stores sell *first-aid kits* as a unit, or you can buy the following items separately:

- Six to 12 sterile gauze pads of 2, 3, and 4 inches square.
- Sealed gauze roller bandages 1, 2 and 3 inches wide.
- Assorted sizes of adhesive strip bandages (Band-Aid, Curad, etc.).
- Small roll of adhesive tape, ½ inch wide.
- Roll of sterile absorbent cotton.
- Two slings or 2 pieces of cotton material about 1 yard square that will fold to make a triangular bandage.
- Scissors with rounded ends.

- Pair of small tweezers.
- Selection of large and small safety pins.
- Two thermometers, 1 for mouth and 1 for rectum.
- Flashlight. (Note: use long-life batteries for storage.)
- Box of safety matches.
- Package of needles for removing splinters.
- Tongue depressors.
- Small box of cotton swabs (Q-Tips).
- Four-inch elastic (Ace) bandage for sprained ankle, wrist, elbow.
- Unbreakable bottle of aromatic spirits of ammonia for treating person who feels faint.
- Unbreakable bottle of oil of clove for treating toothaches.
- Soap.
- Unbreakable bottle of alcohol.
- Bottle of household (3 percent) hydrogen peroxide.
- Calamine lotion.
- Razor blade.
- Tourniquet.

You will also want to have on hand the following *first-aid medicines and ointments*. If possible, keep them next to the medical supplies and separate from other medications. But *be sure* to keep all medications out of reach of small children.

- Antiseptic cream, lotion, salve, or spray.
- Two bottles of aspirin, 1 for adults and 1 for children.
- Petroleum jelly.
- Table salt or salt tablets.
- Baking soda.
- Syrup of ipecac.
- An antihistamine.
- Kaopectate.
- Universal antidote, available from a druggist, for poisoning.
- Pepto-Bismol.

WHAT TO DO WHEN YOU ARE INJURED AND ALONE

1. Panic is your worst enemy. Remain calm by praying, talking to yourself, and thinking things through.
2. Decide as quickly and sensibly as possible what is wrong. Is it a heart attack, broken leg, bleeding ulcer?
3. Can you get help? Where is the nearest person, the nearest phone? Can you attract attention by yelling, firing a gun, building a fire?
4. If the problem is an injury (such as a sprain, fracture, laceration, or animal or snake bite), you should be able to bandage or strap it or apply pressure to stop the blood flow. Should you apply a tourniquet? Be sure to use clothing to stop bleeding. If the bleeding is stopped, you probably will have time for the remaining problems.

But if you have sustained a major medical emergency, try to think about procedures you have read or heard about or learned from friends or relatives. Lie down and make yourself as comfortable as possible. Don't get in the way of nature by overexerting yourself. Remember that the human race survived millions of years without hospitals, medicines, or doctors.

SECTION THREE

Care at Home

Home-care situations that need immediate or constant attention.

ABRASIONS

Description: An abrasion is a friction, scraping, or scuffing injury to the skin, as when a person "skins" an elbow or knee. Abrasions are seldom serious, but they are susceptible to infection.

Treatment

- Wash your hands with soap and warm water before treating the injury.
- Wash the affected area with plenty of soap and warm water. If possible, place the wound under a running faucet. Cleanse the wound by using a sterile dressing or a newly laundered cloth.
- If dirt or foreign matter are ground into the abrasion, a lot of cleaning can be done, with only brief pain, by a quick scrub with a brush. Or call a doctor for advice.
- Apply a *mild* antibiotic ointment (Bacimycin or Neosporin are examples) to the wound.
- Then apply a non-sticking dressing or an adhesive bandage strip (Band-Aid, Curad). If neither is available, place some petroleum jelly on the abrasion, then cover it with a sterile gauze pad secured with adhesive tape.
- Leave the dressing in place for 24 hours, making sure it is kept clean and dry.
- For minor abrasions, after 24 hours remove the dressing at night to prevent the area from becoming too moist. Tip: You can remove a dressing without its sticking to the wound by pouring a small amount of household (3 percent) hydrogen peroxide onto the affected area before you pull off the bandage.
- *Be sure* to watch for infection. If pus, pain, redness, swelling, or tenderness increases in the affected area, contact your doctor.

ALLERGIES
and Allergic Reactions

Description: Allergies are abnormal tissue reaction to normally harmless, non-toxic substances (such as chocolate, cosmetics, nuts, shellfish, and strawberries).

NOTE: Swelling in the mouth or on the tongue is always serious because it can interfere with breathing. Immediate medical help is needed.

Three of the most common allergies are asthma, hay fever, and hives.

ASTHMA

The patient has difficulty forcing air out of the lungs, exhaling with a wheezing sound.

Treatment

- Although the asthma attack can be frightening for both the patient and the observer, even acute incidents are seldom serious medical emergencies. The best treatment is to provide reassurance.
- To help the patient return to normal breathing, turn on hot water in a sink or shower and let him breathe in the moist air.
- Consult a doctor who can treat the condition. The doctor may prescribe one or more compounds, which must be administered according to specific instructions. Tests probably will be run to determine the ultimate cause of the asthma attacks.
- It may be necessary to remove the cause from the asthma patient's environment or to remove the patient from the area.

NOTE: Fastest relief comes from injections of various medications, which requires a visit to the doctor's office or nearest hospital.

HAY FEVER

Caused by pollen in the air, this allergic reaction results in an itchy and runny nose, itchy and watering eyes, and sneezing.

Treatment

- Antihistamine pills and nose drops offer some symptomatic relief to hay-fever sufferers.
- Have the patient avoid drafts and wind.
- You might contact a doctor who would administer a "desensitization" treatment. This involves the injection of increasing doses of pollen extracts at various intervals.
- In severe cases of hay fever, some patients move temporarily or permanently to another environment which does not have the offending pollen.

HIVES

Hives are usually caused by a food such as strawberries, peaches, or lobster; or medication such as penicillin. This allergic reaction results in small, usually round bumps, often salmon-pink in color, that are itchy. Hives last from a few minutes up to 24 hours, seldom longer.

Treatment

- Before giving the patient any food or drink, determine the cause of the allergy if possible. It is permissible to give him water.
- In prolonged cases, seek a doctor's advice.
- If you have an antihistamine (such as a hay-fever remedy), give it to the patient. Give other medication *only* upon a doctor's instructions.
- Do *not* let the patient take a hot bath or hot shower, because the *heat* will aggravate the skin's itching and swelling.

NOTE: The patient may begin an allergic reaction. He may start wheezing, and he may show signs of shock. This condition can lead to death. If the patient seems to be getting progressively worse, take him to the nearest hospital.

100

APPENDICITIS

Description: The appendix is a blind tube, measuring from one half to six inches long and about one quarter of an inch in diameter, that is attached to the large bowel in the right side of the lower abdomen. When the appendix becomes infected and inflamed the disease is called appendicitis, and it is serious.

Symptoms

- The victim experiences a "bellyache," generally situated in mid abdomen; the ache gets progressively worse.
- He has no desire for food, develops nausea, often vomits.
- Pain moves to right lower abdomen, where it becomes very sensitive to touch as the disease progresses.
- Pushing in on appendix area is quite painful, but letting go hurts even more.
- Patient usually has 99°–100° F. temperature.

Treatment

- Contact your doctor and explain the symptoms. Follow the doctor's instructions.
- Do *not* give the patient a laxative or an enema.
- Do *not* apply heat to the abdomen.
- But an ice bag placed over the affected area might provide some relief from the symptoms. Of course, the cooling process will not affect the cause.
- The only treatment is prompt surgery, before the appendix ruptures. So, in case an operation is needed, do *not* give the patient any food or drink. It is best that he not have a full stomach when the anesthetic is administered.

ATHLETE'S FOOT

Description: This fungal infection of the foot causes small cracks and sores that appear on the skin, particularly between the toes. It may spread to other parts of the body, where it can cause a rash, and the cracks may become the site for other infections.

Treatment

- Gently wash away the scaly or damp peelings.
- Dry the feet, especially between the toes.
- Apply water mixed with a little rubbing alcohol.
- Dry the feet again.
- Apply a bland dusting powder.
- Expose the feet to the air as much as possible.
- Before bed at night and first thing in the morning, apply a mild fungicidal ointment (such as Desenex).
- Wear absorbent socks.
- If the athlete's foot persists, have the patient see a physician.

102

BACKACHE

Description: There are many forms of back pain, especially aches of the lower back, and there are many conditions and causes. The most common causes of backache are improper lifting of objects, even if they are not heavy, and direct injuries. Other causes include poor posture while walking, standing, or sitting; nervous tension; arthritis; and a slipped disk.

Treatment

- For mild backaches, give the adult patient two aspirin every four hours.
- Apply a heating pad to the affected area, but be sure it is *not* so hot that it burns the skin.
- Have the patient soak in a hot bath.
- Similarly, hot, moist compresses can help relieve the discomfort.
- A firm mattress may be necessary. A bed board or some plywood inserted between the mattress and box spring will help.
- If the pain persists, however, have the patient see a doctor.

BLADDER PAINS

Description: The bladder, which is part of the urinary tract, is a hollow organ with muscular walls in which urine collects before voiding. A number of disorders can affect the bladder, including stones, benign and cancerous tumors, infection, and inflammation.

Symptoms of bladder disorders are pain in the area of the bladder, frequent urination, difficult urination and, often, bloody urine.

Treatment

- Drink lots of water to flush kidneys and bladder.
- Antibiotic medicines usually cure bladder pains and disorders, but these drugs must be prescribed by a doctor.
- *Always* consult a physician about frequent, painful, or difficult urination. Do not attempt to treat these conditions yourself.
- Stones should *not* be treated with home remedies that supposedly "dissolve" them. Instead, have the patient consult a doctor. It may be necessary to have the stones removed by surgery, but most will pass spontaneously.

BLEEDING (MINOR)

(Also see Bleeding [External], pg. 7, and Bleeding [Internal], pg. 12.)

The great majority of abrasions, cuts, and other surface injuries and disorders that produce bleeding are not serious. The main danger is from *infection.*

Treatment for Most Instances of Bleeding

Everyday cuts and scrapes can be treated according to the following:

- Wash the affected area promptly with plenty of soap and warm water. It is best, if possible, to use clean tap water that pours down on the injury while you are cleaning it.
- If you have cleaned the injury properly, there is no need to use an antiseptic. But as long as the antiseptic is not so strong that it causes pain, you may want to apply it.
- Place a sterile dressing over the cut, then fasten the dressing with a bandage. For small abrasions and cuts, an adhesive bandage strip (Band-Aid, Curad) is suitable.

Nosebleeds **(Also see Broken Nose, pg. 156.)**

Most nosebleeds are more annoying than serious. Usually, they merely indicate that a minor blood vessel has ruptured. Exceptions are nosebleeds resulting from a disease such as high blood pressure, which can cause heavy, prolonged, and dangerous bleeding; and nosebleeds resulting from an injury.

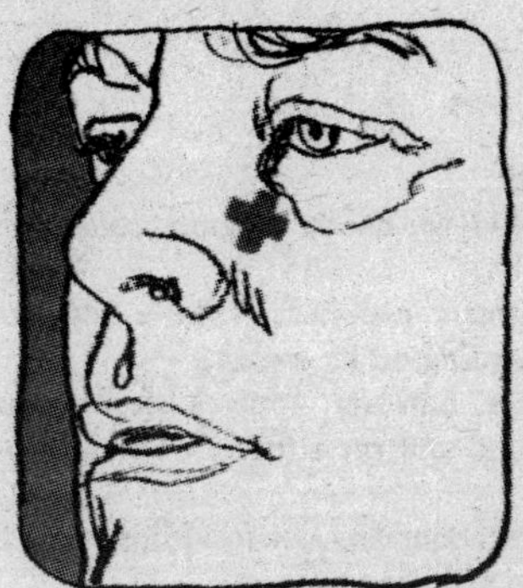

Pressure point.

- Keep the patient quiet. If possible, keep him in a sitting position with the upper body leaning forward. If that is not possible, he should recline with the head and shoulders raised.
- Apply direct pressure to the nostrils by pinching at the soft portion below the hard bone for 10 minutes.
- If the bleeding continues, insert a small pad of sterile gauze (not cotton) into one or both nostrils. Then pinch the nostrils tightly with your thumb and index finger. *Be sure* the sterile pad extends outside the nostril for easy removal (cotton may be hard to remove).
- If bleeding still continues, contact a doctor. The nosebleed is now serious enough for medical attention.

Cut Lips

These common injuries usually are easily treated and fast healing. Be mindful, however, of possible infection.

- Use no antiseptics.
- Instead, wash the affected area gently with soap and warm water. Then apply cold water to help stop the bleeding.
- You can also hold a sterile gauze pad over the wound to help stop the bleeding.
- If the injury is sustained by a child, *be sure* to caution him against biting or touching the wound with his fingers. Otherwise infection is likely.

Cuts Inside the Mouth

- Minor cuts of the tongue, cheek, or gums sometimes bleed heavily then stop completely.
- Seldom is any treatment necessary. Take a few moments to see if the wound stops bleeding on its own.
- If bleeding continues, however, apply a sterile gauze compress or ice cube to the wound and press firmly on it with your thumb and forefinger.
- Consult your doctor about any cut inside the mouth that concerns you because of its size or appearance.

Bleeding from the Ear

Depending upon the cause, this injury may or may not be serious but it needs to be examined by a physician.

- If the bleeding follows a head injury or a blow directly to the ear, *contact medical help immediately.* It may be necessary to rush the victim to a hospital emergency room.
- If pus is mixed with blood, the disorder may be an infection of the middle ear. Apply a sterile gauze pad over the ear, then contact your doctor for advice.
- But if there have been no blows to the head or ear and there is no pus, yet the bleeding continues, suspect a foreign body in the ear. Do *not* try to dislodge the foreign matter yourself. That might cause further injury. Do *not* push cotton into the ear. That might be difficult to remove later. Instead, place a sterile compress over the ear, tell the patient not to touch it, and contact your doctor for advice.

BLISTERS

Description: Blisters are caused by rubbing, or by burning from the sun's rays or other heat which results in a collection of fluid in the outer layer of the skin. Blisters resulting from heat are often serious and should be seen by a doctor. But blisters from rubbing usually can be treated at home.

Treatment

- Wash the affected area with soap and warm water.
- Dry and clean the area with rubbing alcohol.
- Then apply a sterile gauze dressing or adhesive bandage strip over the affected area.
- DO NOT break the blisters.
- Prevent other blisters by having the patient examine hands or feet for "hot spots."
- If found, pad the hot spots with a rubber-adhesive dressing with a hole in the center or with an adhesive strip (Band-Aid, Curad, etc.).

108

HIGH BLOOD PRESSURE

Description: High blood pressure (also called hypertension) is not a disease in itself. But it may be a warning signal of a disease, a result of temporary nervous tension, or it may have no known cause.

This condition occurs when the walls of the arteries constrict, narrowing the space through which the blood must flow. When the space is reduced, the pressure rises.

Symptoms include weakness or exhaustion, headaches, dizziness, or faintness. In its severe form, high blood pressure may cause blurred vision. Very often, people who suffer from high blood pressure have no symptoms at all.

Treatment

- In some cases, dietary restrictions may bring down the pressure. Salt, for example, may have to be eliminated from the diet. Overweight patients may find that weight loss results in reduction of the blood-pressure level.
- There are incidents of high blood pressure as a diagnosis when, in fact, the patient was simply nervous about the results of the blood pressure test. As a result of his nervousness, the pressure level became temporarily high.
- It is always best to have a physician examine a patient who has or may have high blood pressure. Only in that way can an underlying disease, if any, be diagnosed.
- In most cases, the high blood pressure is easily treated with medications prescribed by a doctor. But very often, the patient neglects taking his medicine because high blood pressure has no symptoms. This is very dangerous. Medication must be taken as directed.

BRUISES

Description: Bruises (also called contusions) are usually caused by a fall or a blow. The skin is not broken, but the small blood vessels under the skin are ruptured, resulting in swelling when the blood flows into the surrounding soft tissues. Pain and tenderness to the touch are other accompanying conditions.

The blood that collects is usually absorbed gradually without causing any difficulty. People with light-colored skin will see the bruise change from black and blue to brown to green to yellow.

Treatment usually is not required except to relieve pain.

To Lessen Pain

- Apply ice packs and you will relieve some pain and swelling.
- Or place an absorbent cloth under cold running water, wring it out, then apply it to the bruise.
- If necessary, rest and elevate the injured part.
- But if the bruise is severe and there is a great deal of pain and swelling, contact your doctor.

110

CHILLS

Description: The sensation of being cold, accompanied by shivering and pallor, is termed the chills. In a healthy person, chills are a normal defense against exposure to cold, because the work done by the muscles when shivering produces heat that keeps the body temperature from falling.

However, when followed by fever, chills are a symptom of an infection. A chill is often the first stage, for example, of several acute infections, such as pneumonia, scarlet fever, and influenza. Other causes of chills are toxic substances in the blood or shock following an injury.

Treatment

- Relieve common chills by putting more clothing on the victim, increasing the heat in his room, and giving him warm drinks and warm baths.
- But chills that are accompanied by a general feeling of illness or fever should be brought to the attention of a doctor.

COLDS

(Also see Flu, pg. 133.)

Description: Colds are the most common nuisance diseases. About 90 percent of the people in the United States have at least one cold each year, and most of us have several. "Three days coming, three days with you, and three days going" is an old and often accurate description of the course of colds.

Symptoms include a dry stage, in which the nose feels prickly and there is a tickling sensation in the throat; then the eyes become watery; sneezing, a running nose, a cough, sore throat, headache, and some fever usually follow; and then the secretions become thick and the cold begins to dry up.

Treatment

- Contact your doctor when a person with one of the following conditions or diseases catches a cold: bronchial asthma, chronic bronchitis or bronchiectasis, emphysema, severe diabetes, heart disease that is severe enough to cause shortness of breath, kidney disease, severe liver disease, rheumatic fever, rheumatic heart disease, severe sinusitis, or tuberculosis.
- The otherwise healthy person who comes down with a cold should get plenty of bed rest. Bed is the best place to stay warm, avoid changing temperatures, and prevent contact with others who have not yet caught the cold. It is best if the patient stays in bed until he is past the runny stage of the cold.
- Give the patient plenty of fluids. He may eat moderately any foods that do not cause indigestion.

- *Be sure* to caution the patient against blowing his nose too hard. Otherwise, he will force the infection into the sinuses and ears.
- Patent nose drops may or may not be adequate treatment for a stopped-up nose. You might want to get your doctor's recommendation about nose drops or inhalers.
- Antihistamines may or may not be therapeutic. Again, check with your doctor.
- Aspirin will bring the quickest and safest relief. But relief, of course, is not the same as a cure. There is no cure for the common cold.
- See that the patient smothers all coughs, and sneezes into tissues or handkerchiefs. This action will greatly lessen the spread of infection. And have him wash his hands frequently; infection is often transmitted by hand.
- *Be sure* to call the doctor if any of the following occurs:
    1. The fever lasts for more than three days or goes above 102° F.
    2. the patient has a severe headache that does not respond to aspirin.
    3. Chills, severe cough, chest pains, or blood-stained or rusty-looking sputum accompanies the cold.
    4. The patient aches all over, or aches in the back, neck, or other bones or has earaches.
    5. If the cold symptoms do not clear up, the patient may not have a cold. Instead, he may have hay fever or another allergy. Check with your doctor.

CONGESTION OF THE NOSE

Description: Nasal congestion—a stuffy or runny nose—is a symptom of the common cold and may also be caused by chronic infections, allergies, nasal polyps, or infected adenoids.

Note that nose drops, inhalants, and antihistamine pills do not cure congestion. They suppress the symptoms of colds and other conditions.

Treatment

- Nose drops may be a better treatment for nasal congestion resulting from a cold than are antihistamine pills. Avoid oily nose drops, however, for they have a possibility of dripping into the lungs, where they may cause damage. Nose drops should not be used for more than 3 days.
- Antihistamines are often most useful for treating congestion of the nose related to allergies.
- Decongestant medications shrink the mucous membranes of the nose and therefore widen the air passages. Decongestants are available in tablets, liquids, nose drops, inhalants, and sprays.
- Let your doctor decide whether or not to prescribe any medicine and what kind it should be.

114

CONSTIPATION

Description: Constipation is difficulty in bowel movement. It usually results when the waste material has become compact and hard, making it painful to evacuate. Constipation is rarely serious, unless it is the result of an organic disease. Most often, it is caused by improper diet, nervous tension, insufficient exercise, or overuse of laxatives.

Although one bowel movement every 24 hours is average, many healthy men and women find it normal to have a bowel movement once every 36 or 48 hours. It is possible to become so concerned about the lack of a bowel movement that it is delayed further. If there is no discomfort, there probably is nothing to worry about.

Treatment

- Consider the patient's diet. It should contain roughage, such as leafy green vegetables, fruits, whole-grain cereal, and bread. Dates, figs, and prunes are beneficial too. Fluids and lubricants are essential, including water, milk, fruit juice, and soups.
- Nervous tension often contributes to constipation. Constant worry could indicate the need to talk things out with an interested friend or doctor. A doctor, of course, has additional aids at his disposal.
- The patient can train his body to evacuate regularly. To promote bowel movements after breakfast, for example, he can drink a glass of fruit juice, tea, or coffee before eating. Then, after breakfast he can sit on the toilet for at least 10 minutes, becoming as relaxed and comfortable as possible. He should avoid feeling hurried or tense. With patience, the bowels can be "taught" to move regularly.
- Do *not* give laxatives or cathartics to children; if possible, adults should avoid them too. Laxatives can actually cause constipation.

They are bowel irritants. Regular irritation may result in a bowel becoming less and less sensitive to any stimulation—eventually resulting in constipation. For those adults who cannot take an enema, a mild laxative may be indicated, such as milk of magnesia.

- If constipation persists, consult a doctor to determine the underlying cause.

116

COUGHING

Description: Coughing is an attempt to clear the air passages of anything that causes irritation or blockage. Because coughing serves a useful purpose, it is usually unwise to try to suppress it entirely. Instead, try to determine its cause.

Mucus from the common cold is a most frequent cause; others include smoking and bronchitis. Such serious diseases as whooping cough, emphysema, tuberculosis, and lung cancer may be the underlying condition for which a cough is just a symptom.

Treatment

- If a cough persists for more than a few weeks or if bloody sputum is coughed up, seek a doctor's advice.
- Infants who cough should receive medical attention without delay.
- Because coughing is so common, there are a host of syrups and palliatives available. These substances temporarily relieve a tickle in the throat, but they will not cure a cough, nor will they cure any underlying condition.
- Strong or hacking coughs should be brought to a doctor's attention.
- Antihistamine medications may be taken to dry up secretions.
- If the nose membranes are congested, a vaporizer may bring symptomatic relief. A steaming kettle is an alternative to a vaporizer.
- Hot fluids—milk, cocoa, coffee, or tea—may also help reduce coughing. Many people still get relief with old-fashioned honey, tea, and lemon—with or without a little added whiskey.

117

DIARRHEA

Description: Diarrhea is the frequent, excessive discharge of watery material from the bowel. The chief danger from this condition is loss of too much water, or dehydration. Diarrhea also interferes with nourishment, because digested food passes through the intestine before it can be absorbed into the system.

Possible Causes of Diarrhea Include

1. Eating and drinking too much or too rich food.
2. Eating foods that are contaminated.
3. Allergic reactions.
4. Emotional stress.
5. Swallowing harmful substances.
6. Various infections.

Note below a special discussion of diarrhea in infants, which can be serious.

Treatment

- Mild cases of diarrhea usually can be relieved by readily available remedies, including kaolin-pectin preparations.
- *Be sure* the patient restores fluids to the body by taking liquids such as tea and light soups. Hot drinks are especially helpful after each bowel movement.
- If traveling, diarrhea may be caused by germs that are new to your system. Eat bland foods if they are available, including boiled or poached eggs, custard, and rice with milk and sugar. Water may be contaminated, so it may be best to drink bottled water.

- Some over-the-counter medicines are very effective in relief of diarrhea; Pepto-Bismol is one excellent remedy.
- If diarrhea lasts more than a day or two, consult a doctor.

IMPORTANT: **Diarrhea in Infants**

- Diarrhea in *infants* under two years of age is often more serious than diarrhea in adults, because babies' bodies are tiny and cannot tolerate much fluid loss. Even in mild cases involving infants, *notify your doctor.*
- *Any* major difference in a baby's stools, especially if they contain mucus or blood, is cause for consulting a doctor *immediately.*
- If diarrhea is mild and doctor is not readily available, dilute the baby's usual formula with water to half strength, or use half water and half skim milk. Give it frequently, in small amounts.
- If vomiting accompanies the diarrhea, provide the following formula as a temporary substitute:

  1 quart of boiled water
  2 tablespoons of sugar or corn syrup
  1 level teaspoon of salt (not more).
- *Older children* may be given the same formula. If they refuse it, any clear liquid can be substituted, provided it contains some salt in the proportion of one level teaspoon to one quart.
- These very restricted diets are *temporary measures only.* They should be discontinued after consulting with your doctor or after 24 hours.

SLIPPED DISKS

Description: Disks made of cartilage—the same material that shapes the nose and ears—lie between the bones of the spine. Disks may deteriorate, be injured, or be ruptured thus causing body weight and activity to squeeze a portion of the disk outward to press against the spinal cord or nerve roots emerging from the spinal column.

Pain and disability are common symptoms, often most pronounced in the lower back and made worse when coughing, sneezing, or straining. Later, the pain may spread down one or both legs. Symptoms can come and go, but eventually they may severely handicap activity.

Treatment

- For accurate diagnosis, see a doctor. X-rays and other tests may be required.
- Bed rest on a hard mattress placed over a bed board is often helpful. Later, a surgical corset may be needed or, in the case of a slipped disk in the neck, a special collar may have to be worn.
- Various medications are often helpful.
- Much relief can be obtained from graduated special exercises to strengthen the back muscles.
- In some instances, surgery is necessary.

120

DIZZINESS

Description: Dizziness is used to describe a great variety of sensations, but the main characteristic is a feeling of movement when, in fact, there is none. The patient feels that he is swaying, rocking, pitching, falling, drunk, whirling, or that the room is whirling around him; yet all is still. This whirling sensation is called vertigo.

Severe vertigo is usually the result of a disorder affecting the organs of the inner ear, or the nerve pathways that connect these delicate organs of balance to the brain. Motion sickness and ear wax may produce vertigo. Vascular changes in older people are frequent causes too. Other cases of dizziness may be the result of infections, fever, hypertension, fainting, injuries to the head, viruses, and a variety of diseases. In these instances, the patient may describe the feeling as dizziness or light headedness.

Treatment

- Have the person lie down. Or put him in a semiprone position, if that is more comfortable.
- Be aware that nausea and faintness may accompany the dizziness. If the patient is about to vomit, turn his head to the side so that the vomitus is not inhaled.
- If the attack of dizziness does not pass quickly, contact your doctor.

DRUG ABUSE

(Also see Drug Overdose, pg. 55.)

The following discussion of drug abuse offers more detail than is found in Section One. The information here may help you identify the particular substance, according to the patient's reactions to it, and follow through with specific treatment.

The material is presented in the following order:

1. Alcohol
2. Amphetamines
3. Barbiturates
4. Hallucinogens
5. Inhalants
6. Narcotics (Narcotics by definition are drugs that in moderate doses dull the senses, relieve pain, or induce sleep, but in excessive doses cause stupor, coma, or death.)

ALCOHOL

Alcohol is a sedative, or depressant, that acts strongly on the central nervous system to impair coordination, interfere with judgment, and remove inhibitions. It is never a stimulant.

Signs and symptoms of alcohol abuse often include:

- Hilarity
- Joviality
- Anger
- Truculence

- Agitation
- Confusion
- Slurred speech
- Alcoholic breath
- A red face
- Difficulty walking

Further abuse may lead to the patient's turning white, breaking out in a cold sweat, vomiting, drowsiness, and perhaps passing out. Alcohol abuse can result in physical dependence—alcoholism.

Treatment

- There is not much you can do to treat a person who is under the influence of alcohol. Giving him strong coffee and inducing vomiting really doesn't do very much. It is best to try to keep him calm, stop him from driving or operating any kind of machinery, and get him to sleep it off.
- *Help* is what is really needed for someone who frequently abuses alcohol. There are many organizations set up to help the victim of alcoholism. The most well known is Alcoholics Anonymous; or call your local hospital if you feel you need the name of a center or clinic for chronic patients.
- But if a member of your family is an alcoholic, what he or she is doing to you can be as bad as the effects on himself. Al-Anon is an organization for the families of alcoholics. Consult your telephone directory for more information.

AMPHETAMINES

Amphetamines are stimulants that have the opposite effect on the nervous system to depressants such as alcohol and barbiturates. Amphetamines are sometimes prescribed to curb the appetite of dieters, combat fatigue, or reduce mild cases of depression.

Common names for amphetamines include uppers, bennies, diet pills, and pep pills. The best-known examples of these pills are amphetamine sulfate (marketed as Benzedrine ®) and dextroamphetamine sulfate (Dexedrine ®).

Signs of Amphetamine Abuse

- Jitters
- Unclear speech
- Irritability
- Tension
- Dulled emotions
- An inability to organize thinking
- Loss of appetite and weight.

The pupils become dilated, the mouth often is dry, there is sweating (especially of the palms of the hands), and there may be headache, nausea, and paleness. Amphetamine abuse does not cause physical dependence but may cause psychological dependence.

SPEED is the common name for a related stimulant, methamphetamine hydrochloride (Methedrine ®) and Desoxyn ®). Speed may be injected intravenously and can cause hallucinations, paranoia, and suicidal impulses.

Treatment for Amphetamine Abuse

- Give the patient emotional support in a quiet, reassuring environment. Offer understanding and encouragement to counteract his possible lack of emotional control.
- If the patient has taken an overdose, call a doctor. The physician may administer special drugs to act as an antidote.
- Psychological counseling may be necessary.

BARBITURATES

Like alcohol, barbiturates are sedatives. Barbiturates are prescribed to relax the central nervous system, as in the form of sleeping pills, for example.

Some of the Medical Names of Barbiturates Include

1. Pentobarbital (Nembutal ®)
2. Secobarbital (Seconal ®)
3. Phenobarbital (Luminal ®)
4. Sodium amobarbital (Amytal ®)
5. Sodium butabarbital (Butisol ®)

These pills are sometimes called barbs, downers, yellows, pinks, phennies, and other names.

Signs of Barbiturate Abuse

- Mental confusion
- Loss of emotional control
- Staggering
- Stumbling
- Drowsiness
- No scent of alcohol on the breath.

Because the body develops a tolerance to barbiturates, the dose must be continually increased to get the desired effect. Barbiturates are physically and psychologically addicting. An overdose can lead to coma and death. When combined with alcohol, the depressant effect of each drug is enhanced, *increasing* the risk of an overdose.

HALLUCINOGENS

The most popular hallucinogen, marijuana, is hallucinogenic only in large doses. Hashish is similar to and more powerful than marijuana and is prepared from the same hemp plant. Far stronger forms of hallucinogens include lysergic acid diethylamide (LSD), mescaline, and psilocybin, which are also called psychedelic drugs.

Marijuana is often called grass, pot, Mary Jane, reefers, and many other names. It is usually smoked, giving off a pungent odor much like burning rope. Symptoms include hilarity, euphoria, disorientation as to time, impairment of judgment, and some mental confusion. Increased perception, leading to allegedly greater insight into art and music, is often claimed. Hallucinations are rare. Marijuana does not cause physical dependence, but it does have a potential for psychological dependence.

LSD (known as acid), mescaline (mescal or peyote), psilocybin (magic mushroom), as well as dimethyltryptamine (DMT), phencyclidine (PCP), and dimethoxy-4-methylamphetamine (STP), are usually ingested in tablets or capsules or saturated in sugar cubes and eaten. All of these substances produce hallucinations that can cause exhilarating sensations (a good trip) or depression and severe fright (a bad trip). Symptoms include marked changes in everyday behavior, dilation of pupils, and increased body temperature.

Sometimes the abuser of hallucinogens believes he has superhuman abilities, such as flying, that can encourage him to take dangerous risks. Continued use may lead to psychological dependence. An overdose can cause serious mental changes.

Treatment for Hallucinogen Abuse

- There is no specific treatment for abuse of marijuana. Emotional support is usually sufficient until the substance has worn off.
- Emotional support is far more critical in response to the abuse of the stronger hallucinogens. Sometimes it is possible to talk the user down off his high and thereby calm his fears.
- Contact emergency medical help.
- Always protect him from hurting himself and others and from being injured by objects in his immediate environment. If possible, take the patient to a quiet, safe room. Stay with him.
- A bad trip can be ended by the use of counteracting drugs, which must be administered by a doctor.

INHALANTS

Inhalants are chemicals that are sniffed to get "high." Sniffing the glue used to build model airplanes and toys is the most popular example.

Other substances that are inhaled include nail-polish remover, gasoline, lacquer, paint thinner, and various aerosol sprays.

Symptoms include:
- Drowsiness
- Inability to talk clearly
- Clumsiness
- Memory loss
- Watery eyes
- The odor of the substance on the breath and clothes.

Prolonged or repeated inhalation causes damage, especially to lungs, brain, liver, and kidneys, and there is a potential for psychological dependence. Death by suffocation is a possibility for the abuser who passes out with his head inside a bag or sack containing the substance.

Treatment for Inhalant Abuse

- Immediately get the victim away from the chemical source.
- Check to see if the victim is breathing adequately. If not, give him artificial respiration (see pg. 29).
- Make sure any victim of inhalant abuse has plenty of fresh air.
- Have someone contact a doctor.
- Treat the patient for shock (see pg. 79).

NARCOTICS

Heroin, morphine, and opium are pain-killers that are strong depressants of the central nervous system. Codeine is another narcotic, but it is not nearly as powerful. Heroin (also called snow, stuff, H, and junk) is the most often abused narcotic. These substances usually are injected with a hypodermic needle, though they can be sniffed, too.

Two medications, Demerol ® and Percodan ®, are frequently prescribed to counteract moderate to severe pain but are commonly abused drugs. So is Methadone, which is used legally under certain circumstances in the maintenance of narcotics addicts.

Cocaine, a narcotic, is a stimulant that can be sniffed (snorted) in powdered form, injected in liquid form, or taken by mouth to achieve a brief state of exhilaration. Sometimes called coke, this substance can cause psychological but not physical dependence. An overdose can lead to death. Cocaine abuse frequently produces paranoia and thus makes the abuser dangerous to others.

Symptoms of narcotic abuse include a "high" characterized by easing of fears and relief from all cares. Tiny pupils and scars or puncture marks on the arms are common. The use of hypodermic needles carries with it the possibility of contracting hepatitis and tetanus. Heroin, morphine, and opium are both psychologically and physically addicting.

Treatment for Narcotic Abuse

- Make sure the patient is breathing adequately. Be prepared to give him artificial respiration (see pg. 29).
- Have someone get medical help. Narcotics are one of the few toxic chemicals for which a specific antidote is available.
- Treat the victim for shock (see pg. 79).

TRANQUILIZERS

Tranquilizers also are sedatives. They are prescribed to provide a calming effect on the central nervous system. Some commonly used and abused tranquilizers are Librium, Valium, and Miltown.

Treatment for Barbiturate and Tranquilizer Abuse

- If the patient is conscious and the substance was ingested within the past 1–2 hours, induce vomiting. Wash out the stomach as much as possible by giving him large amounts of water, then encourage further vomiting.

NOTE: If the substance was ingested more than 4 hours before, little of the drug is likely to be retrieved by vomiting. And there is the danger that a semicomatose patient will inhale the vomitus into his lungs. Therefore, in this case do *not* induce vomiting.

- If the patient is conscious or easily aroused, he may be fine but should be closely observed.
- However, if the victim becomes unconscious, *be sure* to maintain breathing. Artificial respiration may be required (see pg. 29).
- After breathing is maintained in the unconscious patient, treat him for shock (see pg. 79).
- Have someone contact medical help. The unconscious patient must be transported to a hospital.

EARACHES

(Also see Foreign Object in Ear, pg. 130.)

Description: Painful sensations in the ear most often are produced by infections, which usually cause high fever in children.

In addition to pain and fever, a third symptom is partial or complete but temporary deafness in the affected ear. An infant with an earache will continually rub or pull at the infected ear.

Treatment

- Call your doctor. Let an authority advise you about proper treatment. If an infection is the cause, the doctor may prescribe an antibiotic.
- Use ear drops *only* with your doctor's advice.
- Do *not* put heated oil into the ear.
- Do *not* wash the ear out with a syringe.
- Do *not* poke into the ear canal with a cotton swab or any other object.
- For less than severe earaches, provide aspirin (see label for dosage).
- A heating pad or a hot-water bag placed over the ear may provide additional comfort.

FOREIGN OBJECT IN EAR

(Also see Earaches, pg. 129.)

Foreign bodies such as insects sometimes fly into ears. And children often put such objects as beads or seeds into their ears.

Treatment

- *Never* poke any object into the ear in an attempt to dislodge the foreign material; you may perforate the delicate eardrum. The safest procedure is to have a doctor remove the object.
- If you are *sure* that the ear problem is caused by an insect and not an infection or other foreign object, you might proceed as follows. Pull backward a little on the top of the ear to straighten the ear canal. While the patient's head is turned to the opposite side, fill the canal with some warm olive oil, mineral oil, or baby oil. The oil drowns the insect and prevents it from biting the canal or drum. After a few minutes, the patient will know that the insect has stopped moving. Flush the ear canal gently with warm water until oil and insect are washed out.
- Other foreign objects are treated differently, so it is best to seek professional treatment.

BLACK EYE

Description: A minor blow near the eye often produces a bruise. Minute blood vessels beneath the skin have ruptured, resulting in discoloration and swelling. Because of the number of blood vessels and the transparency of the skin in this area, the bruise is darker than it would be elsewhere.

Treatment

- Reduce the pain and swelling by immediately applying ice packs or cloths soaked in cold water and wrung out.
- Inspect the eye. Contact a doctor if the eyeball appears damaged (bloody, the patient cannot see well, or the pupil is different from the uninjured side or shows other problems).

SLIGHT FEVER

(Also see Fever, pg. 66.)

A fever that is about 100° F. by mouth or 101° F. by rectum is not usually considered serious. As you know, however, a fever is a symptom of a disease or infection, so even a slight fever should be treated and watched with care.

Check for nasal congestion, sore throat, cough, scratchy throat, and other signs of cold or illness. Nausea, chills, and rashes may be signs of more serious sickness.

Treatment

- Take and record the temperature.
- Then give aspirin, Tylenol, or similar medication.
- Record the temperature every four hours and note the severity of any other symptoms.
- Have the patient get as much rest as possible.
- Contact your doctor if fever lasts more than 1–2 days.

FLU

(Also see Colds, pg. 111.)

Description: Also called influenza and the grippe, flu is an acute infectious disease caused by a virus. (Intestinal flu is a non-medical term for several kinds of intestinal upsets that have no connection with the flu.)

Flu symptoms include fever, chills, headache, loss of appetite, general aches and pains, weakness, and inflammation of the mucous membranes of the nose and throat. Because it is often difficult even for a doctor to distinguish between a cold and flu, regard every cold that seems severe or lasts a long time as potential influenza.

Flu virus weakens the body's defenses against bacteria, making the patient susceptible to developing pneumonia caused by secondary infection with one of several kinds of bacteria.

In uncomplicated cases, acute symptoms of flu last only a few days. A general feeling of weakness, however, can hang on for several weeks.

Treatment

- There is no known cure for flu. The best treatment is to have the patient go to bed at the first symptoms, and stay there as long as the acute symptoms last.
- If there are aches and pains, consult your doctor. The physician will prescribe medication to relieve the symptoms, and antibiotics if bacterial infection threatens or has developed.
- Although it is useless to have flu shots after symptoms have developed, an injection of virus vaccine before the onset of this disease might prevent it by offering temporary immunity. After the injection, it takes about two weeks for the immunity to be acquired.
- Temporary immunity also follows recovery from flu, but because there are several strains of this disease, having one kind does *not* immunize the patient from a different strain. It is best, for the patient to gradually return to normal activity with the advice of a doctor.

FOOD POISONING

Food poisoning results from eating bacterially poisoned foods, or from eating plants or animals containing natural poisons.

BACTERIALLY POISONED FOODS

Foods that are contaminated with bacteria are foods that are bacterially poisoned. A physician who knows what food has been eaten and the patient's symptoms often can make a diagnosis. In addition, many times, *several* people are affected by food poisoning, so you may be able to determine the source of contamination by calling people who have been with the victim, or friends and neighbors who shop at the same stores.

There are four major types of bacterially poisoned foods: streptococcal, staphylococcal, salmonella, and botulinus.

Description: *Staphylococcal* food poisoning occurs when certain foods are stored at temperatures that are too warm. Suspect foods include all kinds of processed meats (especially cold cuts), dairy products, and cream and custard pies. Symptoms, which occur a few hours after eating, include nausea, vomiting, abdominal pain, and diarrhea. Fever is rare. But note that the victim may appear to have the grippe or the intestinal grippe.

Treatment of Staphylococcal Food Poisoning

- Be prepared to help the victim combat shock (see pg. 79). Although the intestinal pain can be severe, this form of food poisoning seldom causes death. Shock is often the most serious result.

Description: *Streptococcal* food poisoning is caused by bacteria in cream-filled pastries, dressings in meat and fowl, and canned foods or leftovers that have not been recooked. Colic, diarrhea, nausea, and vomiting will occur about four hours after eating the infected food.

Treatment of Streptococcal Food Poisoning

- Make the victim as comfortable as possible.
- Give him liquids and bland, soft foods only.
- In most cases, do *not* try to stop the diarrhea, because that is the body's way of trying to eliminate the toxin. But if the victim is too uncomfortable, give him a little paregoric.
- In severe cases, contact your doctor.
- Contact a doctor, who might administer certain sulfonamides or antibiotics.

Description: *Salmonella* food poisoning can involve almost any food. The sources of contamination may be diseased animals, droppings from animals and insects, or the handling of food by a human carrier who may or may not show any symptoms. Very often, several people are affected by salmonella food poisoning.

Symptoms appear after an incubation period of about 6–48 hours and include feeling chilled, nausea, abdominal cramps, and severe and watery diarrhea. The acute aspects of the illness last one to two days, leaving the victim weak for some time.

Treatment for Salmonella Food Poisoning

- Make the victim as comfortable as possible.
- Give victim liquids and bland, soft solids only.
- In most cases, do *not* try to stop the diarrhea, because that is the body's way of trying to eliminate the toxin. But if the patient is too uncomfortable, give him a little paregoric.
- Contact your doctor in severe cases.

Description: Botulism, Clostridium botulinum, is the most serious type of food poisoning. The species of bacteria that causes botulism is a naturally occurring organism that may be present in all vegetables. When the vegetables are improperly washed and canned, the botulism germs grow and multiply and secrete an extremely potent poison. Home-canned vegetables, particularly string beans, are the most common offenders. The botulinus toxin can be destroyed by heat. For example, you can boil the contents of a suspect can for 20 minutes before serving.

Symptoms of botulism occur between 12 and 48 hours after ingestion. Dimness of vision, then double vision, difficulty in talking and swallowing, and paralysis of the throat muscles may become evident. The victim may choke on food when he unsuccessfully tries to swallow. Death results from strangulation or heart failure.

Treatment of Botulism

- Contact a doctor as soon as botulism is suspected. The doctor will administer an antitoxin.
- Recovery is prolonged. Expert medical and nursing care are necessary.

NATURALLY POISONOUS PLANTS

Poisoning from plants that are toxic by nature occurs less frequently than the bacterial type. The items that are of major concern are poisonous mushrooms, and a variety of attractive berries which children may eat. Chemically contaminated fruits, vegetables, packaged products, etc. are another potential problem.

Symptoms include violent abdominal pain and, often, vomiting, diarrhea, and profuse sweating. But the symptoms depend on the particular poison that is eaten.

Treatment for Suspected Plant Poisoning

- Contact a physician at once or transport the victim to the emergency room of a hospital.
- Be prepared to treat the victim for shock (see pg. 79).
- Watch the victim's breathing, and be prepared to administer artificial respiration if necessary (see pg. 29).

NOTE: Any incident of food poisoning should be reported to your local department of health by your doctor or hospital. Bring a sample of the suspected plant or food. If the cause might be a product traded in interstate commerce, the U. S. Food and Drug Administration should also be notified. The source of the toxin can then be traced and corrected. However, this is a task for your doctor, hospital or local health department, not of the patient or family.

GONORRHEA

(Also see Syphilis, pg. 165.)

Description: Gonorrhea is the most widespread venereal disease in th United States. This highly contagious disease is transmitted during sex ual intercourse or other sexual contact. Blindness can result if the bacte ria get into the eyes of infants during their passage through the birt canal of an infected mother. (To prevent blindness in infants, disinfectan is placed in their eyes.)

In addition to causing pain and discomfort, gonorrhea can lead tc sterility and arthritis in men and women. It also can cause many disor ders of the reproductive system.

Symptoms in men usually appear 3–7 days after exposure:
1. The male patient feels pain when he urinates.
2. There is usually a discharge of pus from the penis.

Symptoms in women are slower to appear and are often absent:
1. Pus may be discharged from the vagina.
2. A burning sensation may be felt during urination.
3. The abdomen may be painful.

If not arrested, the disease may spread into the urinary and reproductive systems of both males and females.

Treatment

- Many antibiotics are effective in curing gonorrhea. A physician is the best person to test for this disease and to administer treatment.

NOTE: Successful treatment of gonorrhea does *not* produce an immunity to the disease. The patient is just as susceptible to later infection as anyone else who might come in contact with gonorrheal germs.

HEAD INJURIES (NO BLEEDING)

(For more information, see Index.)

Head injuries in children are common, and usually are not serious. You will want to observe the child closely, however, to see if there are symptoms of concussions or fractures. Treatment for a minor bump on the head is the same for both adult and child.

Treatment

- If the patient has been rendered unconscious, even for a moment, *be sure* to contact a doctor. This patient should see a physician.
- If the patient has not been knocked out, watch him closely for the next 24 hours. If he vomits, becomes unusually drowsy, or cannot be awakened when sleeping, call your doctor.

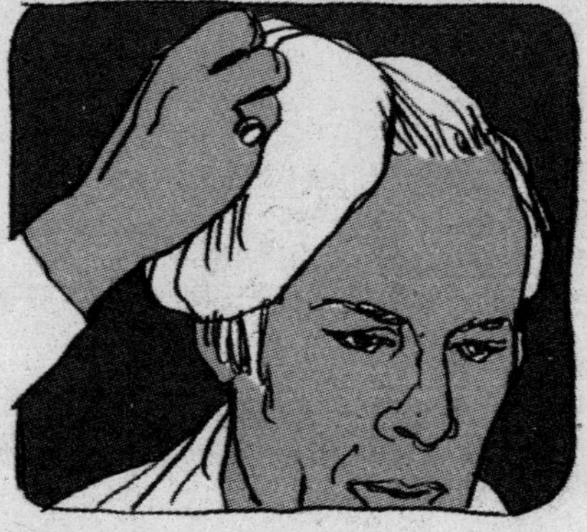

- Any swelling can be lessened by applying an ice pack or a towel soaked in cold water and wrung dry.
- Aspirin and some rest may help speed recovery.

HEADACHES

The pain of headaches varies greatly in type, intensity, and cause. We will discuss headaches according to five groups: common, serious, migraine, tension, and as a symptom.

Common Headaches

Almost everyone has occasional headaches.

- Give the patient aspirin or aspirin substitute (see label for dosage).
- Perhaps have the patient take a warm bath.
- A cold compress on the forehead and another at the base of the skull will provide some relief.
- And bed rest will help the patient somewhat.

Serious Headaches

Get medical help when any of the following occur:

- A head injury leads to headaches.
- A headache is accompanied by stiff neck.
- A headache is sudden, severe, and accompanied by nausea or vomiting.
- A severe headache is accompanied by fever.
- The patient lapses into unconsciousness. *Make sure* he is breathing adequately; if not, give artificial respiration (see pg. 29) and have someone get medical help.

Migraine Headaches

Although the cause of migraine headaches is unknown, certain conditions precipitate the attacks: overwork, fatigue, worry, and stress. Tense people are sometimes predisposed to migraines, as a result of individual psychological factors or a family tendency toward these attacks. In women, migraine headaches often coincide with the menses.

Symptoms vary widely, but a typical migraine headache begins with changes in the field of vision: a flickering before the eyes, flashes of light, or a partial blacking out of vision. These attacks almost never involve the entire head; instead, they are usually confined to one side. Nausea and vomiting often accompany migraine headaches.

- Because symptoms in migraine headaches vary widely, specialists—such as neurologists—are often consulted.
- Aspirin will not help relieve the pain.
- The best treatment is administered by a physician. And sometimes psychological counseling is necessary.

Tension Headaches

Tension headaches are not the result of a disease or any other physical cause. In some cases, they are produced by tension-inducing situations. In other cases, they result more from psychological factors. And lastly, they can be caused by a combination of environmental and psychological factors.

- Aspirin usually will help relieve some of the pain.
- Have the patient rest in a quiet place.
- Applying an ice pack to his head may help too.
- So can a gentle massage of the neck muscles, the temples, and the entire scalp.
- The psychological factors involved in tension headaches may indicate the need for the patient to talk out problems with a psychologist or someone else with special training.

Headaches as a Symptom

- Infectious diseases often show themselves first through headaches. Fever and a general ill feeling frequently accompany head pains in conditions that range from flu and measles to meningitis and even polio.
- Colds, fever, hay fever, and allergies can cause sinusitis, in which membranes of the nose swell, blocking the sinuses and creating pressure that may lead to a headache. The head will throb painfully, especially when the patient leans forward.
- Problems related to high blood pressure, menstruation, and menopause also may cause headaches.
- More serious but less common are brain tumors, which result in headaches that grow more and more painful and are accompanied by a blurring of vision and vomiting.
- Headaches can result from hunger, cold, heat, lack of sleep, overexertion, too much alcohol, too much smoking, anemia, intestinal disorders, and more.

Because headaches can be symptoms of serious diseases as well as common and fleeting maladies, the following guidelines may help you determine whether or not to contact your doctor:

1. If you correct what you think is the cause of the headache but the patient complains of continued pain, you need a doctor's advice.
2. Other symptoms of illness—such as fever, nausea, vomiting, aches and pains—indicate a condition that may be serious.
3. Frequent headaches or those that increase in intensity or duration indicate the need for a medical opinion.

HEAT CRAMPS

(Also see Heatstroke, pg. 72, and Heat Exhaustion, pg. 144.)

Description: Heat cramps are a minor emergency that often, but not always, precedes heat exhaustion. During heat cramps, the muscles tense or spasm. In most cases, the muscles of the arms or legs are the first affected; abdominal pain can also occur. The cause of heat cramps is loss of body water and possibly loss of body salt as well.

Treatment

- To help relieve the spasm, press your hands firmly on the cramped muscles. Or gently massage them.
- Give the patient sips of salt water—½ teaspoon of salt per glass of water.
- Also, have the victim drink plenty of plain water.

HEAT EXHAUSTION

(Also see Heat Cramps, pg. 143 and Heatstroke, pg. 72.)

Description: Heat exhaustion usually is a minor emergency caused by lack of salt. Although the victim's temperature will be about normal, his skin will be pale and clammy. He will sweat profusely, be tired and weak, have a headache, and be dizzy; he might have cramps, become nauseous, and he could faint.

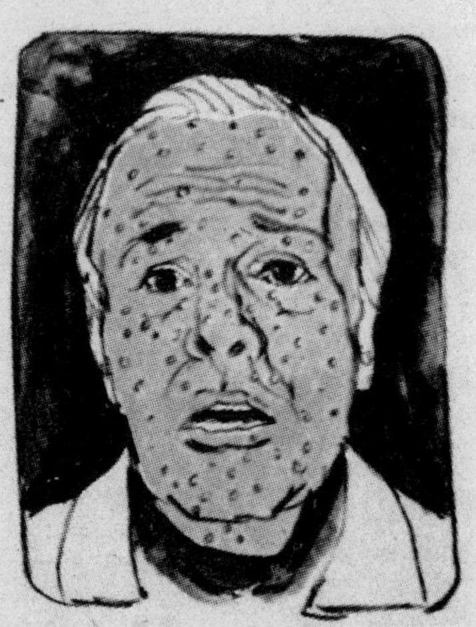

Treatment

- Give the patient sips of salt water (1/2 teaspoon of salt per glass).
- But if he vomits, give no fluids. Take him to a hospital for an intravenous salt solution.
- If he doesn't vomit, have him lie down, then raise his feet about 8–12 inches.
- Loosen any tight clothing.
- Apply cool, wet compresses. Fan him or take him to an air-conditioned room.
- Also, have the victim drink plenty of plain water.

HERNIA

Description: Sometimes known as a rupture, a hernia occurs when there is a weakening or tearing of connective or supporting tissue surrounding an organ, and a portion of the organ bulges through. There are many different types of hernias. The most frequent hernias occur when a loop of intestine protrudes through the wall of the abdomen at either the umbilicus or the groin.

Symptoms include a bulge under the skin (called a hernia sac) that is visible when the patient stands, coughs, or strains. When the patient reclines, the intestine falls back into the abdominal cavity and the bulge usually disappears. If the bulge doesn't disappear, the intestine is caught in the sac. If the intestine then rotates or twists, shutting off the blood supply to that portion of the bowel, this is called a strangulated hernia, and an emergency operation is necessary.

Hernias usually require medical attention.

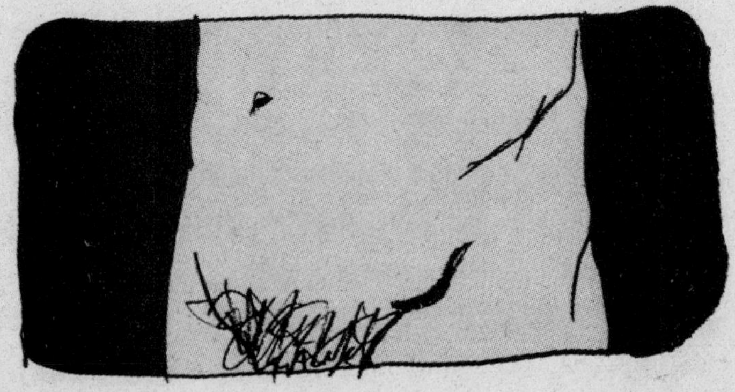

Caution: *Never* press on the hernia bulge, attempting to force it back into the abdomen. The path seldom is straight, and the force might damage the bowel.

Treatment

- Have the patient lie down on his back with a pillow under his buttocks. Soak a washcloth in cold water, wring it out, and apply it gently to the affected area.
- The patient can lie on his abdomen and bring his knees up under his chest so that his buttocks are high. But if this provides no comfort, have him simply lie on his back.
- Get medical aid as soon as possible.

INGROWN TOENAIL

Description: The sides of an ingrown toenail curve into the flesh instead of growing straight out. Not only is this painful; if an ingrown toenail is not treated, it can cause an infection.

Treatment

- If the toenail is only slightly ingrown insert a small piece of cotton under the edge of the nail. Change daily and try to gradually force the nail to grow up and out.
- Protect the nail from pressure by applying a pad of clean gauze around it.
- If the nail is badly ingrown, however, the patient should be seen by a doctor or a podiatrist.

Prevent ingrown toenails from recurring by cutting toenails short, leaving the sides a little longer than the middle. Shoes should be roomy enough so that they do not press on the top or sides of the toes.

MENTAL DISTURBANCES

Mental and emotional illnesses include a great many disorders, most of which are not fully understood. Physical diseases or injuries that involve brain impairment are critical factors in some cases. In other instances, functional disorders are apparent but are not caused by organic brain damage.

Generally speaking, there are three broad classifications of mental disturbance: emotional maladjustment, neurosis, and psychosis.

Emotional maladjustment affects many people from time to time with feelings of moodiness and dissatisfaction, the inability to form satisfying relationships or to hold a job, and/or a tendency to drink too much.

The maladjusted individual may function reasonably well in society, but he is subject to periodic depressions. And sometimes his "personal problems" are complicated by psychosomatic illnesses, which are emotional in origin and show themselves physically.

Neurosis sometimes prohibits the individual from functioning normally. Although he may be able to get by, he usually is unable to relate normally to others on an emotional level.

The neurotic individual may suffer from anxiety, phobia, and/or depression. If he is anxious, he feels fearful and threatened, even though these feelings are basically groundless. He may suffer from a phobia, such as a morbid fear of germs, falling, sickness, crowds, death, or something else. Depression that is prolonged or intense will show itself in pessimism, apathy, and constant fatigue.

Psychosis is far more severe than emotional maladjustment or neurosis. The psychotic individual needs regular psychiatric attention and is often confined to a mental hospital. The psychosis may be organic in origin, resulting from alcoholism, hardening of the arteries, or brain injury. Other forms are generally thought to be nonorganic, including paranoia, schizophrenia, and manic-depressive psychosis.

Treatment for this wide range of mental disturbances varies greatly, of course. In mild forms of emotional maladjustment, a sympathetic friend can be of great help. But most forms of neurosis and all types of psychosis should be handled by specially trained personnel.

The following suggestions may help you provide assistance to an individual experiencing an emotional disturbance:

- Help the person by listening to him. His feelings most likely will include a lack of self-confidence, low self-esteem, and a fear of failure. Some sympathy regarding his problems, some boosting of his ego, and some mention of his strengths and achievements will assist him. Your calmness and encouragement will help him to apply more thought and less emotion to the situation.
- For more serious mental disturbances, try to contact the person's doctor. If that's not possible, get in touch with a close relative.
- If the individual might hurt himself or someone else, call the police.
- Treat the person with respect and patience. He may talk, he may be silent; he may be cooperative or combative; he may be reserved or he may be hysterical. His moods and actions may change. You should try to be a stabilizing influence.
- *Never* argue with him. You can't win, and you might get hurt.
- *Never* state or even imply that you think he is mentally disturbed. That might enrage him.
- To gain his cooperation, be kind and reassuring. Try, also, to be firm without being authoritarian.
- If he is about to commit a rash or harmful act, divert his attention. Get him to think of some other person, object, or idea. If you know who or what he likes, try to bring him around to that subject. Get him to shift his thinking from destructive to constructive acts.
- *Only* if it's absolutely necessary should you physically restrain him. For example, if he is about to injure himself or someone else. It's always best to have someone help you restrain him. You will be more likely to succeed, and you will have a witness to what you did and why you did it.

MUSCLE CRAMPS

Description: Muscle cramps are a form of muscle spasm, one in which the muscle remains rigid for some time. These cramps frequently occur while swimming or during sleep, and they can be extremely painful. They are usually caused by strain, cold, or impaired circulation and fatigue.

Treatment

- Have the person walk around to relieve the cramp.
- Massaging the muscle might help it relax.
- Provide a warm compress or bath.
- If the person has frequent muscle cramps, have him see a doctor.

NAUSEA AND VOMITING

Description: Nausea, a feeling of queasiness in the stomach, and *vomiting,* the throwing up of material from the stomach through the mouth, can result from various causes. Some potentially serious disorders include brain damage, shock, poisoning, and head injuries. Other possible causes include pregnancy, motion sickness, viruses, and flu. Almost all the diseases of the abdominal organs may be accompanied by nausea and vomiting.

Treatment

- Patients who vomit persistently or with great force need *immediate medical attention* to determine the cause of the disorder and institute proper treatment.
- If the victim is unconscious or seriously injured, the main threat is that he might inhale vomitus into his lungs. To prevent this, turn him on his side so that the vomitus or any secretions will flow harmlessly from his mouth.
- For patients who vomit only once or twice, give nothing by mouth for a few hours and wait to see what develops.

Motion sickness:

ONE EXCEPTION IS VOMITING AS A RESULT OF MOTION SICKNESS.

Treatment

- The patient might be given a medication (Dramamine or Benadryl, for example) that is readily available at pharmacies.
- If the patient becomes thirsty, give him small sips of water or a teaspoon of chopped ice, then wait 20 minutes to see if it stays down, before repeating.

- Prevent motion sickness by having the individual eat lightly before and during the trip, thus avoiding an empty stomach, which can contribute to a nauseous feeling. Giving the person Dramamine or Benadryl before the trip can prove effective. So can adjusting the ventilation to get plenty of fresh air. Also, if possible, have him lie flat on his stomach with no view of the scenery and a decrease in his view of the motion.
- When nausea is predictable, it can be lessened by having the person eat lightly of bland foods—perhaps as many as six times per day—such as dry crackers, plain baked potato, whole-wheat bread, and whole-wheat cereal. After eating these solid foods, the patient may sip weak tea, water, or another bland fluid. He should get as much rest as possible, especially after meals. Have him avoid the following: greasy foods, butter, fat, cucumbers, cabbage, cauliflower, spinach, and onions.

NECK INJURIES

Description: Neck injuries can range from minor disorders to those that threaten life. Blows to the front of the neck are particularly dangerous, because tissue damage can cause fluids to drain into the air passages, blocking the airway; extensive swelling can have the same effects. Other neck injuries can involve lacerations and puncture wounds, which can result in profuse bleeding.

Treatment

- Any neck injury has the potential of producing a fracture or dislocation of the cervical vertebra. Most often, when this occurs the body is paralyzed from the neck down. However, in a small percentage of neck injuries, a fracture or dislocation occurs without paralysis. These patients run a severe risk of becoming paralyzed. Thus, when the neck is injured, the head and neck must be properly immobilized before moving the patient.

  Significant neck injuries require an emergency ambulance with the proper equipment to immobilize the head and neck.
- Immediately treat any neck wound that hampers breathing. If the airway is blocked, give the victim artificial respiration (see pg. 29).
- If breathing is interfered with, have someone get medical help while you attend to the victim.

Bleeding from the neck is difficult to control:

- Apply direct pressure to the wound, but *be careful* not to obstruct breathing.
- Extensive bleeding also requires medical attention. But while you assist the victim, have someone else get professional help.
- Keep the victim's head and shoulders raised and the airway free of foreign matter.

- Keep pressure on the wound until medical help arrives.
- *If bleeding is not a problem,* cover the wound with a sterile dressing held in place with tape.
- *Never* apply a bandage all around the neck. Obviously, it could interfere with breathing.

BROKEN NOSE

(Also see Nosebleed, pg. 104.)

A broken or fractured nose can result from a hard blow or by walking into a door or other hard object. Many broken noses go unrecognized. If not repaired soon after injury, serious deformity may result, especially in children. Disfigurement is only one problem; more important, the deformity may obstruct the nasal passages.

Treatment

- Any blow to the nose that causes profuse bleeding should lead to examination.
- Do *not* attempt to splint the fracture.
- If there is bleeding from the broken nose, treat it as a nosebleed (see, pg. 104).
- If there is also an external wound, wash it gently with soap and warm water.
- Apply a soft protective compress. No further covering is needed.
- Provide an ice pack to relieve pain and swelling.
- Take the victim to a physician or hospital for examination.

PARALYSIS

Description: Paralysis is the partial or complete loss of the power to move the muscles in one or more parts of the body. It is alarming, but it is also a useful clue to the nature, extent, and location of an injury or disease.

There are many causes of partial or complete paralysis; mechanical injury, stroke, multiple sclerosis, tumors, and infections of the nervous system are the most common physical causes. Hysterical paralysis is also quite common.

Mechanical injuries occur when the skull or backbone cannot withstand a hard blow, such as during an auto accident. Injury to the brain or spinal cord may lead to paralysis.

A paralytic stroke may result from a blood clot that blocks an artery or from a rupture of an artery in the brain. When this cuts off the blood supply to a portion of the brain, the body parts controlled by that section of the brain are paralyzed. (Also see Stroke, pg. 79.)

Multiple sclerosis, for example, is one of many neurological diseases that strikes the nerves of the brain or spinal cord. Hard patches form on the nerve coverings, interfering with the action of the nerves and resulting in sudden or gradual paralysis in a leg or other part of the body.

Tumors of the brain or spinal column may bring on paralysis because of pressure on sensitive nerve tissue. X-ray treatment may slow the growth of some tumors, and surgery to remove the tumor may be appropriate.

Infections of the nervous system include poliomyelitis (also called infantile paralysis) and spinal meningitis, which damage the spinal cord. Vaccines have been developed to prevent the paralysis caused by poliomyelitis and meningitis.

Syphilis is another infectious disease that, in its advanced stage, attacks the nervous system. Syphilis may result in paralysis and insanity (see Syphilis, pg. 165).

Treatment

- In all cases of partial or complete paralysis, immediately contact medical personnel.
- If the patient is conscious, try to reassure him, and tell him that help is on the way. If the patient realizes that part or all of his body is paralyzed, explain that it may simply be a temporary condition.
- Keep the patient lying on the *affected* side. This allows fluids or vomitus to drain without choking and also allows use of the unaffected arm and leg.
- But if the patient is delirious or combative, it may be more advantageous to lie him on the unaffected side, thus limiting his ability to punch or kick.
- Do whatever you can to help the patient relax. Be prepared to treat him for shock (see pg. 79).

RASHES

Description: Rashes are a temporary skin eruption that may indicate mild disorders such as diaper rash, prickly heat rash, and hives, to more serious illnesses such as chicken pox, measles, and scarlet fever. Allergies, too, are often indicated by rashes.

Because there are so many different possible causes of rashes, there is no general treatment. The following steps may be taken, however, to ease the patient's discomfort.

Treatment

- If the itching is bothersome, put a cup of baking soda in bath water, then bathe the patient.
- Antihistimines often relieve the itching.
- Or you may want to apply calamine lotion to the affected area.
- If the rash persists, or if there are symptoms of illness—such as fever, sore throat, running nose, or general malaise—contact a doctor.

SCRATCHES

Description: Scratches and other small cuts, including those made by cats, dogs, other pets, and people should be thoroughly cleansed to prevent infection.

Treatment

- Take sterile cotton or a freshly laundered washcloth, dip it in warm soapy water, and gently cleanse the minor wound. Remove all signs of foreign matter from the scratch or cut.
- Rinse the wound with plain warm water, preferably by letting tap water run over it.
- If you like, you can apply some antiseptic fluid or cream, but it is not necessary.
- Cover with a sterile gauze pad or a single-strip adhesive bandage (Band-Aid, Curad, etc.).

SORE THROATS

Description: Inflammation and soreness may affect any and all parts of the throat. A sore throat may be the beginning and the end of a minor irritation, or it may be one of the first symptoms of an acute infection, including the common cold, flu, diphtheria, strep throat, infectious mononucleosis, measles, tonsillitis, etc. It may also be caused by smoking, air pollution, and voice strain.

Treatment

- Gargling may provide some comfort. Two crushed aspirin in a glass one-third full of warm water can be effective.
- If the sore throat continues for days, and especially if other symptoms accompany it (fever, headaches, etc.), contact your doctor.

SPLINTERS

Description: Splinters in the hand and other parts of the body are common with both children and adults. These small slivers of wood can be removed fairly easily at home.

Treatment

- Sterilize a large needle by holding it in the flame of a match or by boiling it in water.
- Let the needle cool, but do not let it touch any non-sterile object.
- Sterilize the skin surrounding the splinter by washing the area with warm soapy water. Or dip sterile cotton into some alcohol and rub the cotton gently over the skin.
- Press the point of the needle against the skin. Dig and gently scrape under the splinter until it is loosened or removed.
- If the splinter is partly exposed, remove it with a pair of tweezers that have first been sterilized in alcohol.
- Wash the area thoroughly with soap and warm water.
- Apply a Band-Aid.

NOTE: Dirty puncture wounds, such as those caused by splinters, may need tetanus boosters if the last tetanus shot was more than five years ago.

SPRAINS

(Also see Strains, pg. 164.)

Description: Sprains result when a violent wrenching of a joint causes a tearing of the supporting ligaments. Sprains are more serious than strains, the pain is likely to be more intense, and the affected area will swell because of damage to the surrounding tissues and blood vessels. Most sprains occur in the ankles, knees, fingers, wrists, or shoulders and are caused by falls or athletics.

Note that it is sometimes hard to tell the difference between a sprain and a fracture (see pg. 14). In many cases of apparent sprains, the bones around the joints are cracked.

Treatment

- Immobilize the injured joint with a splint, or with an adhesive bandage or an elastic bandage. Be careful, however, to allow for swelling in the affected area. Check the bandage every now and then to be sure it is not *too tight.* (If around an ankle, the extending foot should be warm to the touch and the skin should be pink, not blue.)
- If possible, elevate the injured part. This will help reduce the victim's pain and swelling.
- You can also reduce pain and swelling by applying an ice pack or cloths dipped in cold water and wrung out. Also, aspirin may help.
- Contact a doctor, because the injury may include a fracture, and the patient may need to be examined by a physician.

STRAINS

Description: Strains occur when muscles and their tendons have been stretched due to overexertion. For example, the muscle fibers may be injured by taking a wrong step and stretching a muscle that supports the ankle. More serious strains involve back muscles that are overexerted because the person has attempted to lift too much weight or has lifted an object improperly. (Remember, lift with your legs, *not* your back.)

Treatment

- Have the patient rest the affected muscles by going to bed.
- Lightly massage the muscles.
- Apply heat with warm, wet towels, hot-water bottles, heating pads, or heating lamps.
- The patient with a back strain will benefit, also, from a board under the mattress for firm support.
- Aspirin may help to reduce pain.
- All severe back strains should be examined by a physician.

SYPHILIS

(Also see Gonorrhea, pg. 138.)

Description: Syphilis is a venereal disease that can cause brain damage, insanity, and death. It is the most serious of all venereal diseases and is transmitted by sexual contact.

There are three stages in this disease:
1. A hard sore (also called a chancre) appears, during the first stage, at the point of contact, usually the genitals. It will eventually heal, even if it goes untreated.
2. In the second stage, 6–10 weeks after exposure to syphilis, a general skin rash appears. Sores on the genitals and in the mouth may be present, and the central nervous system and eyes may be involved too. Symptoms may disappear temporarily, until severe complications appear with stage three. The sores and rashes of both stages 1 and 2 are contagious.
3. But stage three may not be apparent for several years, Skin lesions and tumors may occur, as may syphilitic heart disease, blindness, and other disorders.

NOTE: It is very rare that the female shows any physical symptoms of stage 1 of the disease before it has become seriously advanced.

Treatment

- Penicillin is the main treatment; if it is administered in the first and second stages, syphilis can be cured.
- But note that syphilis can be contracted again and again. There is no vaccine that gives immunity against it.
- The individual who might have syphilis should see a doctor for an examination specifically for this disease. A regular physical examination will not test for syphilis or gonorrhea.

TONSILLITIS

Description: Tonsillitis is not one single disease but a sign of several infectious diseases, including strep throat and diphtheria. Many young children get tonsillitis after their first year, and the onset may be both severe and abrupt.

Symptoms include high fever, up to 104° F. (which may cause convulsions), vomiting, headache, chills, a sore neck, and aching joints. The most important sign, however, relates to the throat: It will be acutely sore, and the patient will have difficulty swallowing.

One look at the throat will reveal tonsils that are enlarged and inflamed. They may be covered with a membrane of pus or with spots that are dirty yellow in color.

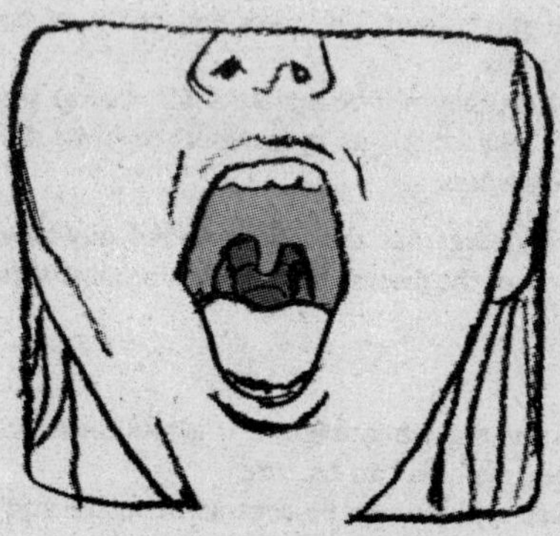

Tonsils enlarged and inflamed.

Treatment

- Contact your doctor.
- If you cannot get the patient to the doctor, some temporary relief may be obtained by placing either hot or cold compresses around the patient's throat.
- For patients who are old enough to gargle, supply a glass of warm water with 1 teaspoon of salt dissolved in it.
- Have the patient stay in bed in a room that is warm and slightly humid, and drink lots of liquids.
- Take aspirin or an aspirin substitute every four hours for pain and fever.

TOOTHACHE

Any persistent pain in a tooth should be examined by a dentist so that permanent relief can be provided. In the meantime, the following should offer temporary pain relief.

Treatment

- Give the patient aspirin or another mild pain-killer. Ice applied to the tooth and gum may be helpful too.
- Heat, however, should *not* be applied to a painful tooth, on the chance that there is a serious abcess. If that's the case, the heat could spread the infection.
- If the toothache is due to a cavity or the loss of a filling, put some oil of clove on a tiny piece of cotton. Then pack the cotton into the cavity with a toothpick or the sharpened end of a wooden match.

169

ULCERS OF THE STOMACH

Description: An ulcer is an inflamed, open sore that can be found in the stomach, the duodenum (a part of the small intestines) or on parts of the skin.

Peptic ulcers occur in the stomach and duodenum and cause severe pain, which worsens when the stomach is empty. Nausea and vomiting may be present also. If untreated, complications (for example, perforation or bleeding) eventually require emergency medical action. Vomiting of blood or "coffee grounds," or passing bloody, black or tarry stools is an urgent sign to get the patient to the hospital.

Treatment

- There is no quick, simple cure for a peptic ulcer. Temporary relief of symptoms is possible by having the patient eat enough to fill the stomach, drink milk, or take an antacid.
- Long-lasting treatment requires careful control of the patient's diet, usually with frequent snacks of bland foods and milk. Spicy foods must be avoided, as should alcohol, tobacco, tea, and coffee.
- Medical care is needed. The doctor may prescribe drugs to neutralize the acidity of the gastric juices.
- Because ulcers usually develop in people who are tense and anxious, efforts should be made to relieve the strain that causes this disorder. Barbiturates and other sedatives may be prescribed to relieve emotional tension. Psychological counseling also may be useful. Environmental changes may have to be made too, to help the patient relax and avoid worry.

SECTION FOUR

First Aid Away from Home

The most common accidents and emergencies that may be encountered while traveling, camping, and engaging in sports and recreational activities.

When taking a trip by car or hiking in the country, you will want to be prepared for special medical emergencies. This section has information about auto accidents, cold-weather injuries, warm-weather injuries, and bites by insects and reptiles.

Other relevant medical emergencies (such as bites by animals, drowning, and nausea) are found in Sections One and Three.

When traveling away from home by car, take your first-aid kit along with you. Add a wool blanket, too, so you can warm an accident victim or fight an auto fire.

Before hiking for an extended period, assemble a *first-aid kit for the out-of-doors.* Select from the following list those supplies that are appropriate for your hike:

- Six to 12 sterile gauze pads of 2, 3, and 4 inches square.
- Sealed gauze roller bandages, 1, 2, and 3 inches wide.
- Assorted sizes of adhesive strip bandages (Band-Aids, etc.).
- Small roll of adhesive tape, ½ inch wide.
- One sheet of moleskin adhesive (or foam adhesive) for blisters.
- Four-inch elastic (Ace) bandage.
- One sling or 1 square yard of cotton material that will fold to make a triangular bandage.
- Scissors with rounded ends.
- Pair of small tweezers.
- Six medium-size safety pins.
- Snakebite kit (Cutter or other brand), to include rubber suction cup, tourniquet, and razor blade.
- Sunburn lotion.
- Insect repellent.
- Salt tablets, 500 mg. each.
- Halazone tablets, for water purification.

- Baking soda or calamine lotion or rubbing alcohol for insect bites.
- Kwell Cream, for chiggers.
- An antihistamine.

If you are away from civilization during certain major medical emergencies, you may need to make splints for arms and legs or provide various methods of transporting or transferring a patient. The following discussion offers alternative methods of splinting injured limbs and moving an individual according to various situations.

BANDAGING HEAD AND JAW

- First cover wound with a compress. Then tie bandage over it tight enough to stop bleeding.
- The twists of gauze over top of head and under jaw will support a fractured jaw, or hold compresses over facial and jaw wounds.
- The twists around the head should be placed low enough on the back of the head so they will not slip off the top of the head.
- Try not to cover the patients eyes with the dressing unless absolutely necessary.

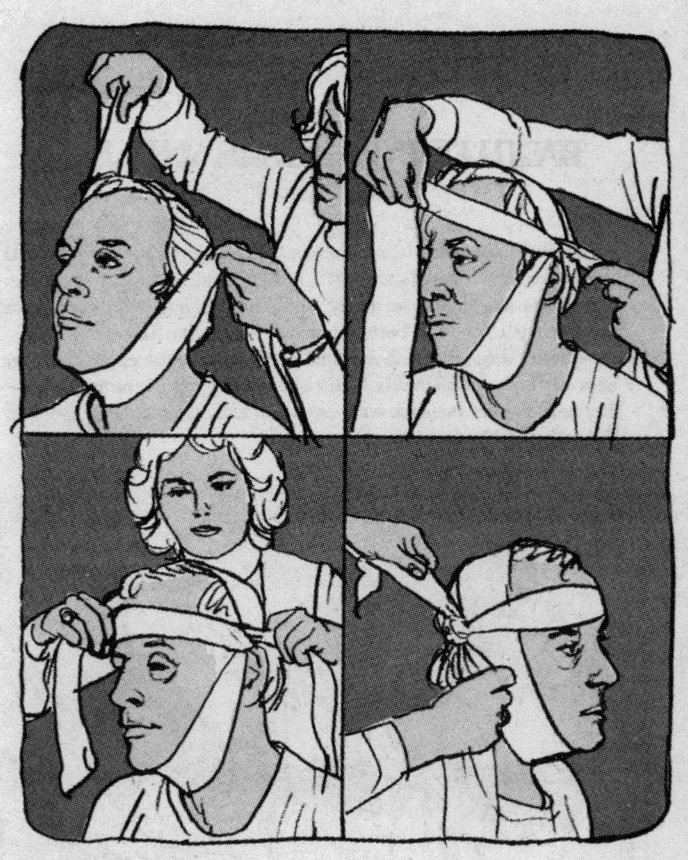

SPLINTS FOR ARMS AND LEGS

- Improvise splints from among several firm objects, including folded newspapers, corrugated cardboard, broom handles, and strong sticks. Materials used should be fairly rigid, strong, and long enough to reach beyond the joint both above and below the fracture.
- *Always* pad the splint with soft materials, such as towels or clothing, to fit the body comfortably while immobilizing the injured part.
- Fasten the splint in place with bandages and strips of adhesive tape or pieces of rope or clothing.

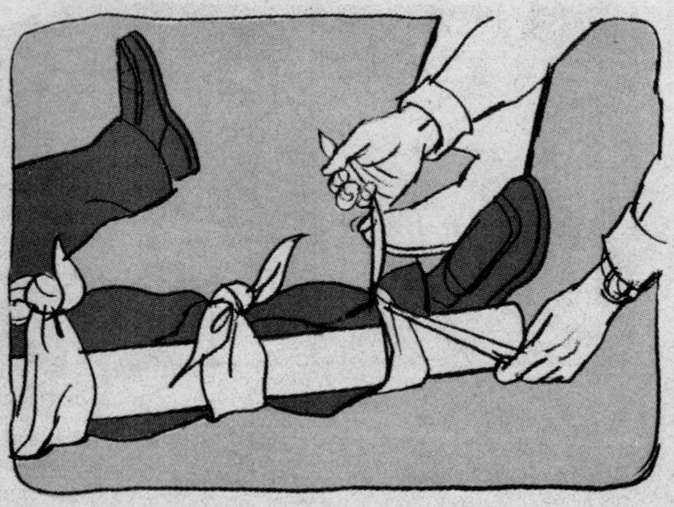

- *Never* make the splint so tight it interferes with blood circulation. If fingers or toes turn blue, for example, immediately loosen the splint. On the other hand, splints should *always* be snug.
- Do *not* allow the splint or fastening materials to pinch the injury.
- If no suitable material is available, use the victim's body to support the injured arm or leg. Tie the injured arm to the body with suitable soft material between the arm and body. Or tie the injured leg to the good leg with padding, such as a blanket or clothing, between them.

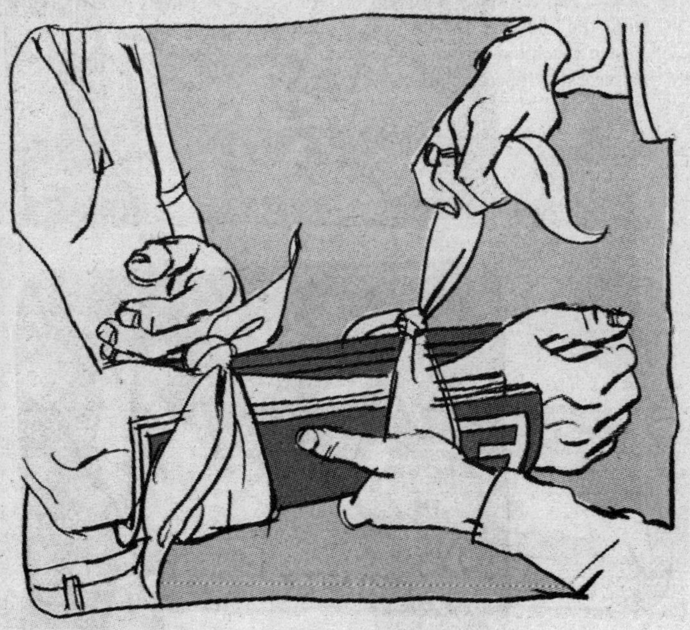

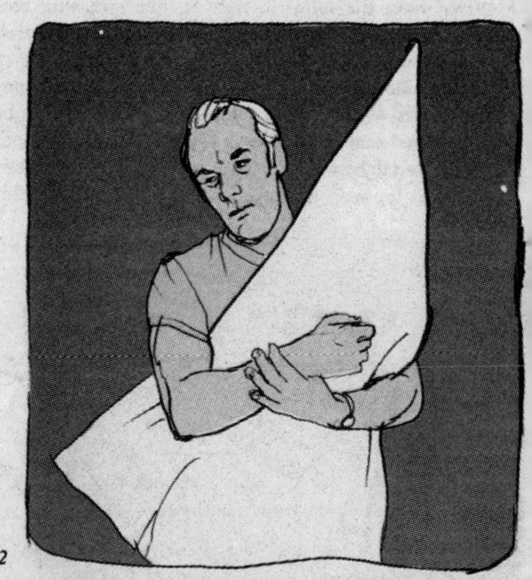

1 & 2

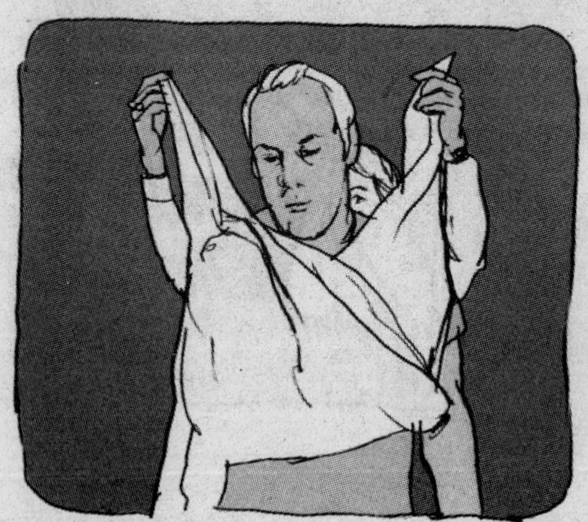

3

How to Make a Sling

1. Use a triangular bandage.
2. Place injured arm over bandage.
3. Bring ends up.
4. Tie behind neck with a secure knot.
5. Pin loose end at elbow.

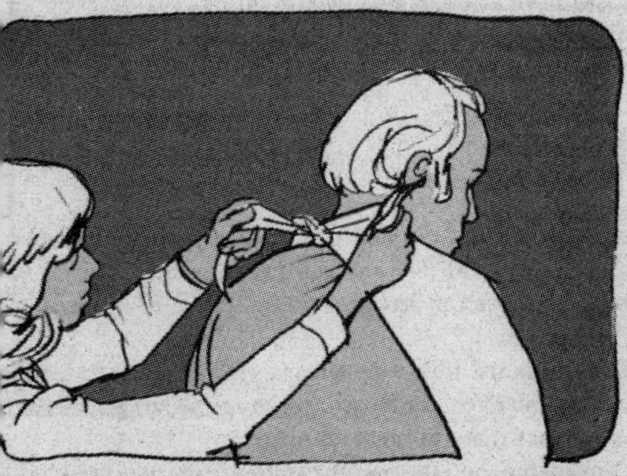

4

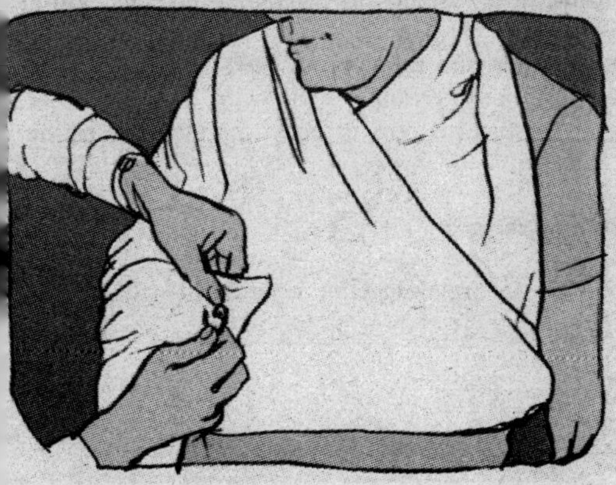

5

METHODS OF TRANSFER

Inexperienced people have a tough time *gently* lifting and carrying an injured person. If there's time, practice on someone else before turning to the injured party.

Pulling a Victim to Safety

- Before you move any victim, *be sure* it is necessary to move him. In many cases, the movement will increase his pain and injury.
- Check to insure that the victim has no injuries of the neck or spine or fractures of any bones.
- When you have determined that it is necessary to move the victim, try to place him on a blanket, cardboard, piece of rug, or large coat. Then, once he's on that material, pull *it,* not him.
- If no material is available, pull or drag the victim from the shoulders, cupping your hands in his armpits. If that is not possible, pull or drag him from the feet.
- Do not pull or drag a victim sideways, as there is a good chance you will increase his injuries greatly.
- Avoid bending or twisting his neck or body, for the same reason.

Supporting a Victim to Safety

- If the victim has no serious wounds or injuries, help him to his feet.

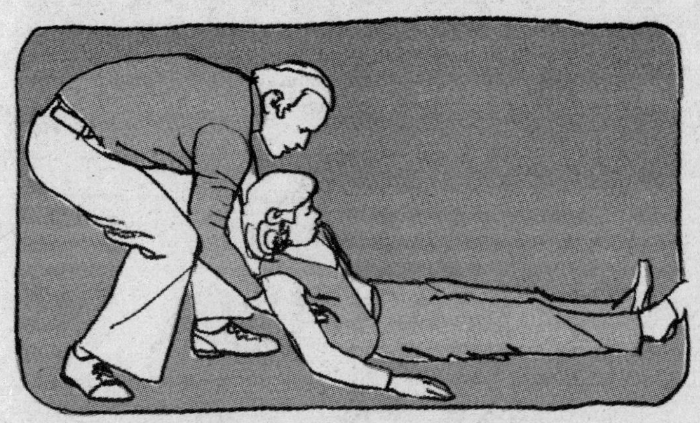

Cup hands under the victim's armpits.

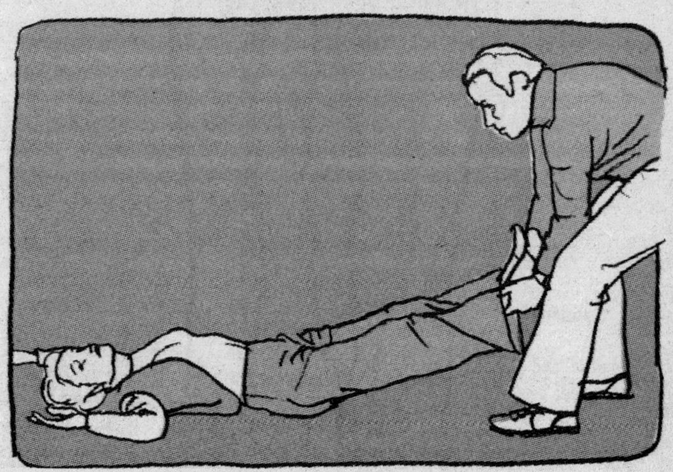

Drag victim by the feet if impossible to pull from the top.

- Place one of his arms around your neck. If a second person is assisting, place the victim's other arm around your assistant's neck. Take hold of the victim's hand as it extends around your neck. Have your assistant do the same with the victim's other hand.
- Place your other hand around the victim's waist, for additional support. Have your assistant do the same.

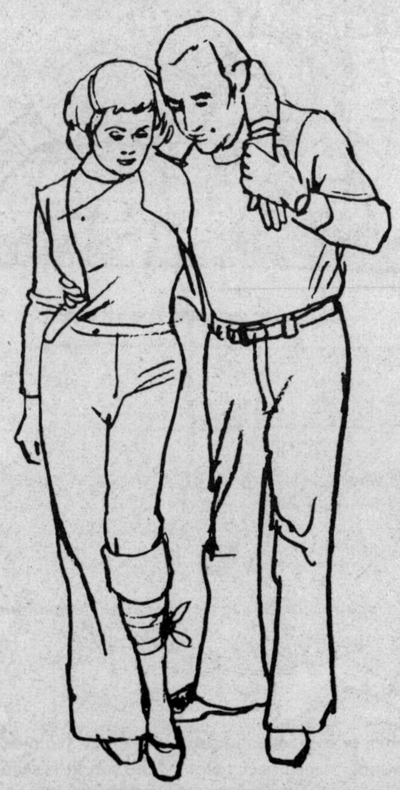

Victim's arm around rescuer's neck.
Rescuer's arm around victim's waist.

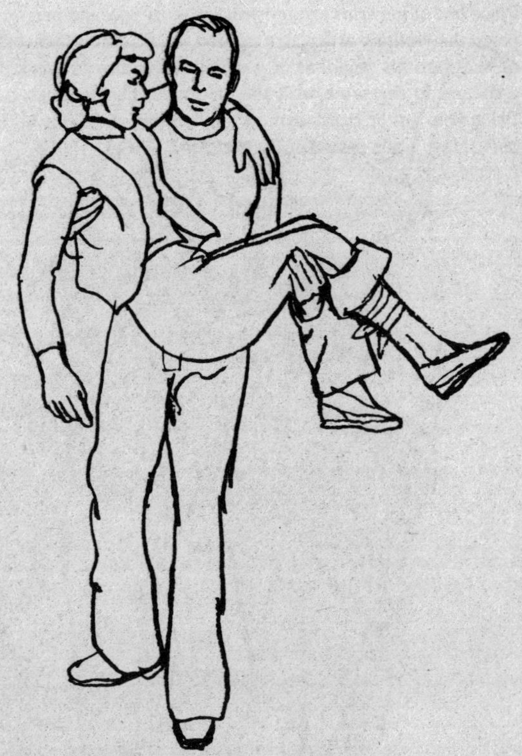

Rescuer's arms under victim's armpits and behind knees.

Improvised Litter

- If no stretcher is available, improvise a litter from a blanket, rug, or heavy clothing placed over poles. Make sure it is secure and sturdy before placing victim on top. Or, if possible, use planks, water skis, floats, or a surfboard. An automobile seat is appropriate for a child.

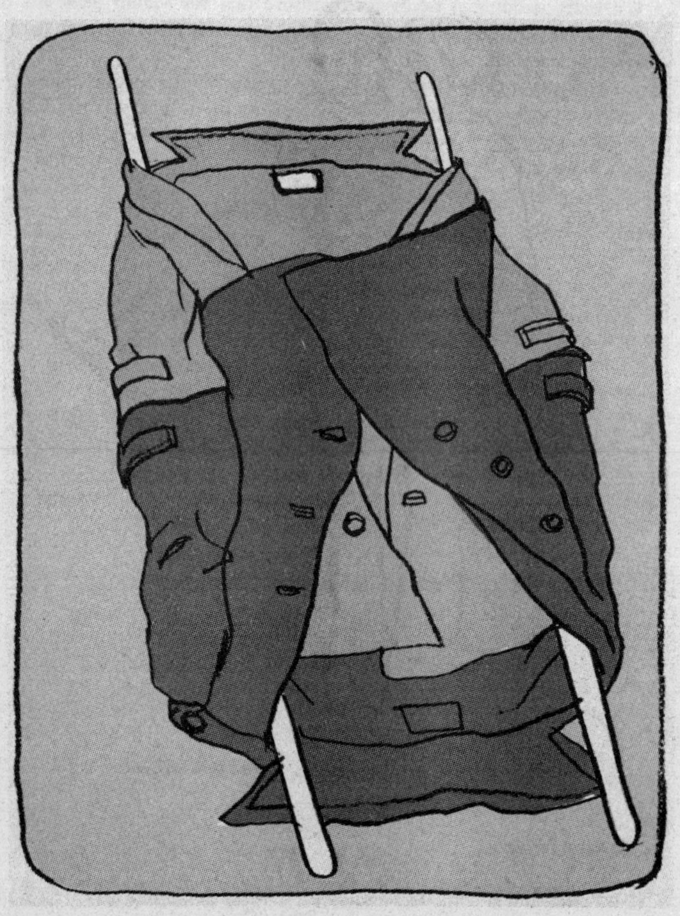

Improvising a litter with coats. Be sure the coats are long enough to support head and feet. Test the litter for strength before placing the victim on top.

- Use extra padding if necessary to insure that the victim does not roll or slide during transit. Give special attention to supporting the victim's head and neck.
- Ideally, you will have four litter bearers. One at the victim's head, one at his feet, and one at either side of the litter. The side bearers will hold the litter with the hand that is closer to the victim. Of course all bearers will face in the same direction and lift the litter at the same time. The minimum number of litter bearers is two.

AUTOMOBILE ACCIDENTS

More than twenty-five *million* Americans are involved in automobile accidents every year. Although most of these are fender benders, several hundred thousand auto accidents cause injuries and fifty thousand cause death.

If you are involved in an auto accident and there are no injuries, you will want to exchange information with the driver of the other car (name, address, driver license number, license plate number, insurance policy number and company, make and model and year of car). Call the police to report all but the most minor instances, and in most cases, contact your insurance company.

In auto accidents where you are not injured or not even involved, assist the victims as follows:

- *Prevent* further injuries. Park your car off the road on the shoulder a safe distance ahead of the accident.
- Prevent fires by turning off the ignition in all involved cars.
- Guard against further accidents by warning traffic. If necessary, start off waving a flashlight, newspaper, or handkerchief to get the drivers' attention. Then, if possible, light flares (but *never* light them near spilled gasoline) and place them 10 feet and 200 feet behind the accident site.
- If there is no highway divider, place additional flares in front of the site.
- If possible, station adults behind the wreckage (in front, too, for undivided highways), to warn traffic. Now that you've acted to prevent further injury, direct your attention to the injured.

1. Have passing motorists call the police.
2. If homes or stores are nearby, send an adult to call emergency services. If possible, do not rely only on passing motorists to contact the police.

3. Have drivers with CB radios in their cars or trucks call for help.
4. *Never* move the injured unless their present position puts them in jeopardy. Any movement may seriously complicate their injuries.
5. Ensure an open airway. If necessary, give artificial respiration (see pg. 29).
6. Control bleeding. Apply direct pressure to the wound (see Bleeding [external], pg. 7).
7. Do whatever you can to make the victims comfortable. Loosen tight clothing, keep them warm—but not hot—by using blankets or coats; keep them lying down.
8. Reassure the victims. Tell them help is on the way. Try to keep them calm.
9. Do *not* let victims walk around. Do everything you can to keep them lying down, even if they say they feel fine. Otherwise they may injure themselves further.
10. *Never* let a victim wander off.
11. Cooperate with emergency personnel when they arrive. Answer their questions. In most cases, you will be on your way in a short time.

BITES BY INSECTS AND PARASITES

Description: Among the most irritating pests in the outdoors are mosquitoes, blackflies, horseflies, and "no-see-ums" (almost invisible flies that exist in warm seasons and have a painful bite).

Prevent bites from these pests by applying liquid preparations containing diethyl toluamide (Off, Mosquitol, Cutter, or 6-12) to hands, face, neck, and other exposed parts of the body. The same ingredient can be sprayed from aerosol cans onto shirt sleeves, trousers, and tent interiors.

Treatment

- Apply ice or cold compresses to the bites or hold them under cold water.
- If possible, make a paste of baking soda moistened with water and apply it to the site.
- Or apply calamine lotion and rubbing alcohol or lotions containing alcohol to help relieve the itching.
- Try to keep the patient from scratching the bite, which could cause infection.

CHIGGERS

Description: These parasites are encountered when walking through grass and low brush in hot, dry areas. They alight on the hiker's pants legs, then find the skin, where they bite and burrow. Chiggers are attracted to tightly constricted areas of the body, such as along the belt line or at the ankles.

Prevent chiggers getting on you by spraying the legs, pants legs, and socks with preparations containing diethyl toluamide (Off, Mosquitol, Cutter, or 6-12).

Treatment

- Destroy the insect with Kwell Creme or a similar preparation.
- Relieve the itching with an ointment containing benzocaine.
- If you have neither of these ointments with you in the wilderness, apply cold wet dressings to the affected area. Treat the condition upon returning to civilization.

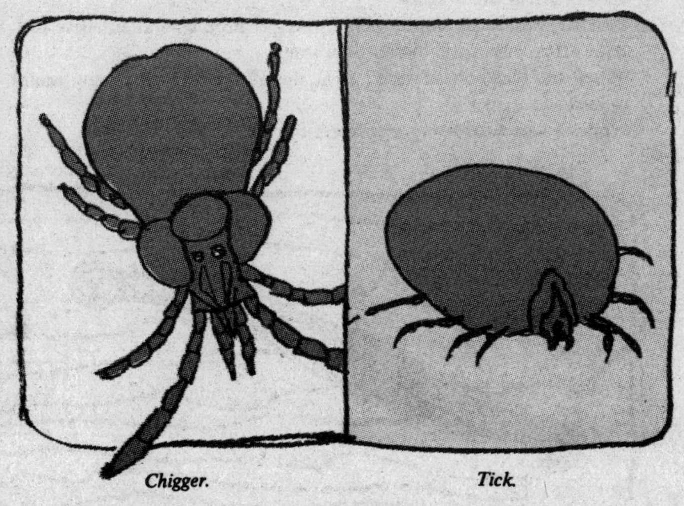

Chigger. *Tick.*

LEECHES

Description: Leeches are small, wormlike, blood-sucking creatures that inhabit relatively stagnant freshwater lakes, ponds, canals, and pools. Leeches may become attached to the skin during wading or swimming. Note that their attachment is painless, however, so the victim often is not aware of them.

Treatment

- When leeches are discovered while the victim is coming out of the water, the creatures can be brushed off easily.
- Once they have been attached for some time, bring the burning end of a cigarette or the coal from a fire close enough to irritate them. They should then disengage themselves.
- Or place a pinch of salt on the leeches, and they will die. Then simply brush them away.
- The skin will bleed quite freely. It may require several adhesive bandage strips before the blood flow stops.
- When the bleeding subsides, treat the affected area like any minor abrasion (see pg. 97).
- Apply a sterile dressing to protect the wound from infection.

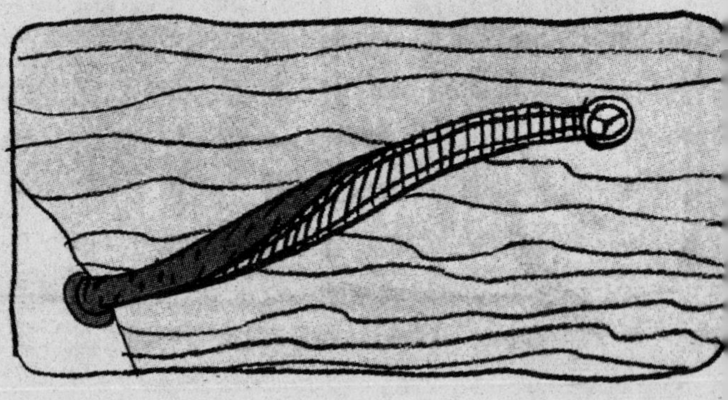

Leech.

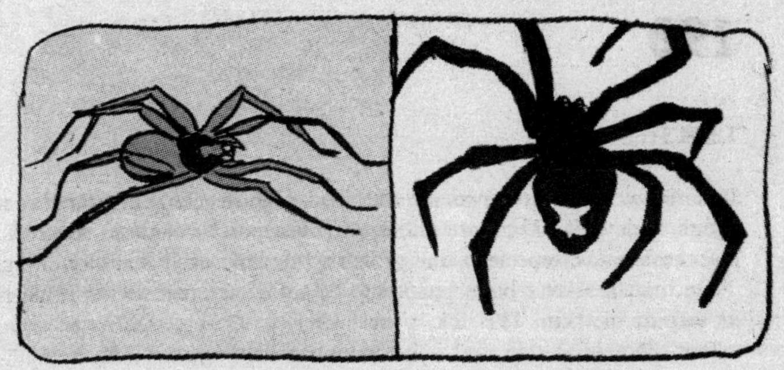

Brown recluse. *Black widow.*

SPIDERS

Description: Almost all spider bites in the United States and Canada are not serious, including those made by tarantulas. The major exception, in wilderness areas, is the female black widow. She is about one half inch long, coal black in color and, on her belly, has a reddish orange mark that's shaped like an hourglass. Also, certain species of brown spiders may cause an ulcerating sore at the site of their bite.

Only the female black widow spider, however, injects a venom that can disable a human. On occasion, children and the elderly die from these bites. Black widow spiders are found in woods, fields, and privies.

Symptoms of black widow spider bites include a sharp pain at the site. The pain may disappear, but about half an hour after the bite occurs, the injected venom causes the abdominal muscles to become rigid. Later there may be difficulty in breathing, tremors, and pain in the limbs.

Treatment

- Examine the skin of the victim for two tiny puncture marks.
- If you find them, get the victim to a doctor as soon as possible.
- Meanwhile, wash the bite with soap and warm water, apply baking-soda compresses, give him coffee as a stimulant, keep him warm and still, and reassure him.
- Be alert for the onset of shock (see pg. 79).

TICKS

Description: These creatures are flat, oval, eight-legged, and about one eighth inch long. They are widespread hazards throughout grass or low-brush areas, especially during late spring and early summer.

Once on a hiker's boot, pants leg, or ankle, the parasite will make its way to the skin. The tick is most likely to attach itself to an area where the skin is thin and offers protective hair growth: the armpit, groin, or buttocks. It will suck many times its body weight of blood, blowing up like a balloon. Then it will drop off.

Ticks can transmit a serious infectious disease, Rocky Mountain spotted fever.

Prevent ticks from attaching themselves to the body by applying large amounts of preparations containing diethyl toluamide (Off, Mosquitol, Cutter, or 6-12). Treat boots, socks, lower legs, and pants cuffs with lotion or an aerosol. It's also best for hikers to pair off and inspect each other for ticks at the end of a day's travel and again first thing in the morning.

How to Remove a Tick

- Do *not squeeze* ticks with your fingers. The parasite's body juices may be infected. Grasp the ticks carefully and remove them with a slow, steady pull. Drop them in a fire or mash them with a rock.
- If the creature remains attached, apply a drop of kerosene or white gas to it.
- Or bring the burning end of a cigarette or an ember from the fire close to the tick, and it will probably disengage itself.
- If it still remains attached, use tweezers to remove it forcibly. Take away its body and as much of its head as possible.
- A portion of its head may remain embedded in the skin. Treat it as if it were a small splinter that cannot be removed. Scrub the area with soap and warm water, then apply a light, sterile dressing.
- If the head festers, scrape it away with the point of a sterilized pin.
- Be alert for fever, chills, or general illness, which may follow a few days after contact with ticks. If these occur, have the patient see a doctor.

EXPOSURE

Description: Exposure is the most treacherous of all types of cold-weather injury. Sometimes referred to as "hypothermia," it is the gradual cooling of the body's inner core to the extent that normal metabolism slows down. Unless the heat loss is discovered and reversed, death will result.

Freezing temperatures are not necessary to cause hypothermia. Dangerous amounts of heat loss can occur between 40° F. and 50° F., especially when accompanied by wind and rain. Psychological factors are also important. The victim who reacts positively to environmental factors and tries to counteract them is likely to survive. The person who panics or despairs is more likely to succumb.

Note that a steady loss of body heat can occur insidiously and become dangerous unless the victim is alert to the threat.

Symptoms of internal body temperature dropping from 99° F. to 97° F. and 96° F. include uncontrollable shivering. When the inner core dips to 92° F. or 91° F., the shivering becomes violent and occurs in waves. The victim has difficulty speaking, his coordination deteriorates, his pace slows, he stumbles, perhaps falls, and his thinking slows. As the body becomes even colder, muscular coordination is seriously impaired and thinking becomes irrational. Pulse and respiration slow, and the victim loses consciousness and dies.

The treatment of exposure involves preventing further heat loss, using external heat sources to warm the body and supplying hot fluids and food to a victim who is conscious.

Treatment

- Provide shelter. The more it keeps out wind and rain or snow, the better, but any shelter is better than none.

- Remove wet clothing and re-dress the victim in dry clothes.
- Get into a sleeping bag and warm it with your body. Then have the victim take your place.
- Or, if the victim is deeply chilled, supply external warmth by having one or more persons huddle up against him inside the sleeping bag. Even better, place sleeping bags underneath and above the group.
- If possible, build a fire near the victim, or build fires on either side of him.
- *Only* if he is conscious, give him hot fluids: soup, coffee, tea, or the like. Fast-energy foods can also do him good: candy and dried fruit are fine.
- The rewarming process may take six to eight hours, depending upon how chilled the victim was. When his body temperature is normal, shivering has stopped, and his mind is clear, move him to medical assistance.
- While moving the victim, *be sure* to keep him warm and dry.

FISHHOOK IN THE FLESH

Treatment depends upon whether or not the fishhook is imbedded in a critical or non-critical area of the body.

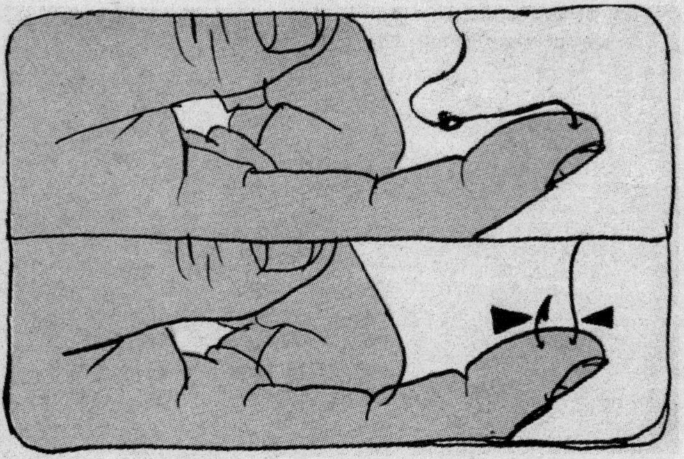

Critical Area of the Body

If the fishhook is in the face or near the eye, or if it has caused a great deal of damage, proceed as follows:

- Cover the wound as is with a sterile dressing.
- Protect it with soft bandaging.
- Have the victim see a doctor as soon as possible.

Non-critical Area of the Body

If the fishhook is imbedded in a finger:

- Expose the barbed end of the hook by pushing it through the skin. If it is not already exposed, press down on the shank of the hook to push the barbed end through the skin. A small cut at the point where the tip will emerge makes this process easier.
- Cut off the barbed end using pliers, wire cutters, etc., then remove the shaft of the hook.
- Wash the wound with soap and warm water. Encourage bleeding.
- Then cover with a sterile dressing.
- A tetanus booster shot may be required if it has been more than five years since the last shot.

FROSTBITE

Description: Frostbite is the most common injury resulting from exposure to the cold. Small areas of the body—the nose, cheeks, ears, fingers, or toes—are usually involved. Frostbite is caused by low temperatures, wind velocity, and type and duration of exposure. Crystals form either superficially or deeply in the fluids and underlying soft tissues of the skin.

Symptoms include *pale and glossy skin;* skin color that changes from natural to white or grayish yellow; pain (may not be present); perhaps blisters; and affected body parts that feel intensely cold. Note that the victim may not be aware that he is frostbitten.

Because body parts actually freeze, advanced stages of frostbite include mental confusion, failing eyesight, unconsciousness, shock, respiratory failure, and death.

Prevention is almost always possible and includes good physical conditioning and adequate food, limiting the length of exposure to the elements, wearing sufficient clothing, and refraining from smoking and alcohol.

Treatment

- *Never* rub or let the patient rub a frostbitten part.
- *Never* apply snow to a frostbitten part.
- When possible, rewarm the affected area *rapidly* by immersing it in water that is between 102° F. and 105° F. If you don't have a thermometer, test the water by dipping your elbow in it, making sure it is just above normal body temperature.
- Rewarming by water will take 20 to 30 minutes and will be accompanied by increasing pain.

- If warm water is not available, wrap the part in warm blankets.
- Do *not* apply hot-water bottles, heat lamps, or heating pads, or place the affected area over a hot fire or stove.

WARNING: Once serious frostbite is treated, the treatment must be complete and the victim must be prevented from contracting the condition again, because a refrozen part is worse off than one that remains frozen. It is better, for example, to let a victim walk for hours on frostbitten feet than to warm the feet, only to have them freeze again, which will make it necessary to carry the patient to civilization and will almost guarantee the need for amputation.

- Thawing of superficial frostbite includes a tingling and burning sensation in the affected area, followed by a purplish or mottled color as blood circulation is restored.
- Once rewarmed, do not allow the patient to use the body part until it has been examined by a doctor. Otherwise tissue damage may be increased.
- Protect the affected area. Keep it clean and warm, as you would keep a burned area.
- Give fluids to a victim who is conscious and not vomiting.

GUNSHOT WOUNDS

Treat gunshot wounds as wounds to a particular part of the body. Penetration of the chest, for example, should be treated as a critical chest wound.

Treatment

- *Always* consider the possibility of fractures, internal bleeding, and internal injuries (see the appropriate discussions in Section One).
- *Never* attempt to remove the bullet from the victim's body. Let the doctor do that.
- Splint a wounded extremity.
- Treat for shock.
- Get the victim to a doctor as soon as possible.

POISON IVY, OAK, AND SUMAC

Description: These plants are found in most sections of the United States and carry an irritating oil on their leaves. When the oil comes in contact with human skin, a chemical and allergic reaction often results, causing intense itching, blistering, weeping of the skin, and swelling of the underlying tissue.

Poison ivy and poison oak are distinguished by leaves that grow in three-leaf clusters. They also have greenish white flowers and berries that grow in clusters. Poison sumac has compound leaves and clusters of small greenish flowers usually followed by hairy fruits.

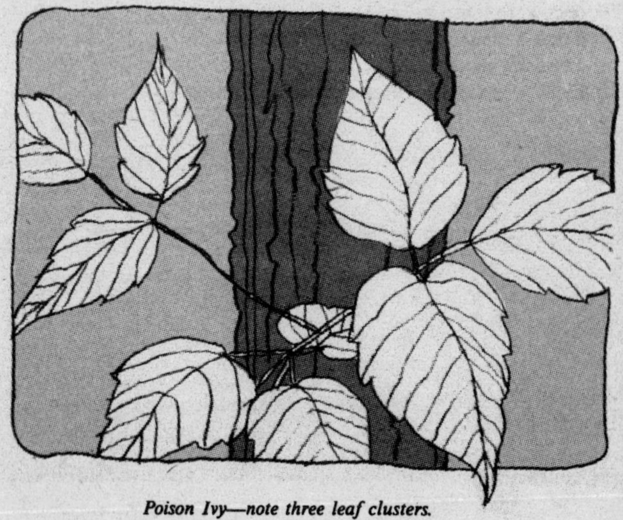

Poison Ivy—note three leaf clusters.

Treatment

- Remove the victim's contaminated clothing.
- Thoroughly wash the exposed area with soap and warm water to remove as much of the irritating oil as possible.
- Apply rubbing alcohol to the affected area.
- If the area is already blistering or itching intensely, apply cold, wet compresses soaked in a saline solution. Dissolve six salt tablets or three teaspoons of salt into a pint of water.
- Or if the affected area is small, itching may be relieved by dissolving two aspirin tablets in a tablespoon of warm water. Then apply the solution as a poultice.
- Mild rashes also may be treated with calamine or other soothing skin lotion.
- An antihistamine may be given to help reduce itching.
- Aspirin will help him get a good night's rest.
- If a severe reaction occurs, seek medical assistance.

SNAKEBITES

Description: There are two types of poisonous snakes in the United States: pit vipers and coral snakes.

Pit vipers include rattlesnakes (found in eastern and western states), water moccasins (which inhibit swampy areas in the South and Southeast), and copperheads (found in fields, woods, and lakes of the Northeast and Middle West). Pit vipers are the most dangerous and will strike without provocation.

Coral snakes inhabit the southwestern United States, as well as southern Texas and Louisiana to Florida, Georgia, and the Carolinas. The toxin in coral-snake venom contains a nerve poison that can cause respiratory failure and widespread paralysis within a few minutes. Coral snakes, however, rarely strike unless provoked. They are brilliantly banded with red, yellow, and black stripes.

Before hiking into wilderness areas, determine which species of poisonous snakes may be encountered, if any, and carry a snakebite kit.

Symptoms of poisonous snakebites often include two puncture marks where the venom has been injected through the fangs, immediate and excruciating pain in the area of the wound, then swelling, generalized weakness, and shock, followed by feelings of suffocation and often prostration. The venom of pit vipers also may cause internal bleeding.

Fast treatment may prevent much of the venom from spreading throughout the victim's body.

Treatment

- Have the victim lie down face upward. Keep him warm.
- Reassure him. Tell him you know what you are doing.
- Apply a tourniquet lightly *above* a wound in an arm or leg. In other words, apply the tourniquet between the heart and the wound. Do

Poisonous snakebite.

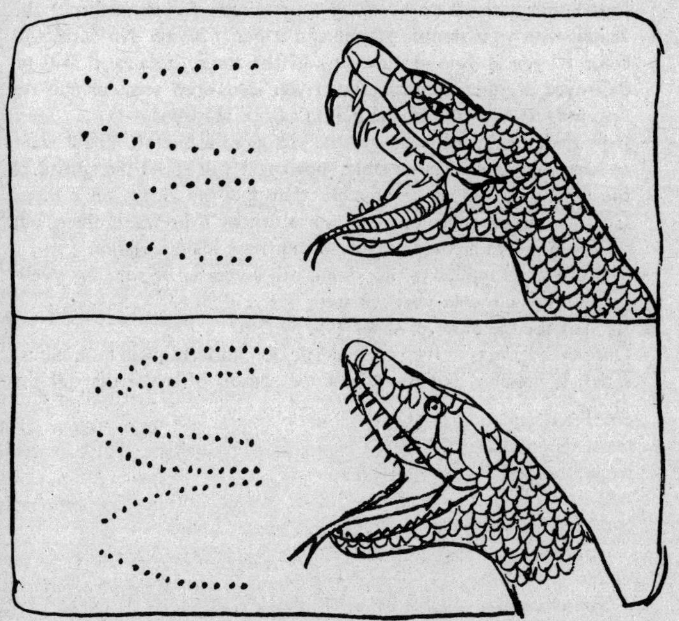

Nonpoisonous snakebite.

not make it tight, because the veins are compressed easily. Use surgical tubing from the snakebite kit, or use a belt, heavy clothing, a bandanna, or a handkerchief.

- Sterilize a knife or the blade of a razor by heating it over a flame. Let the instrument cool without wiping it on anything that is not sterile.
- Then make two ½″ cuts in the victim's skin. Make the cuts parallel to each other, with the punctures between them. (Parallel cuts will heal better than cuts in the form of an X.) The incisions should be only about one eighth inch deep. There is no need to go deeper, or you will cut into blood vessels, nerves, and/or tendons.

- Apply suction to the bite wounds either by using the suction cups in the snakebite kit or by using your mouth. If you suck out the venom with your mouth, simply spit it out. *Caution:* No harm will come to you if you swallow any of the toxin, because it will be destroyed in your stomach. But if you have open sores or cuts on lips, tongue, and cheeks, the poison can be absorbed.
- Now make every effort to get the victim to a doctor. You'll want to keep him as still as possible; movement will speed the spread of the remaining venom. If possible, transport the victim on a litter.
- Give the victim coffee or other warm drinks, if he wants them, but do *not* give him alcohol, which will increase his circulation.
- Wet dressings applied to the wound will decrease the pain and swelling. Do not use cold water or ice.
- Be alert for the onset of shock (see pg. 79).
- Once the victim is in the hands of a doctor, antivenin will be administered. If possible, tell the doctor the species of snake that bit the victim.

STINGS BY BEES, WASPS, AND HORNETS

(Also see Allergic Reactions.)

Description: Bees, wasps, and hornets sting by injecting irritating chemicals into the skin. The resulting lesion may ache or throb for hours.

Treatment

- If the species has left a stinger in the affected area, remove it or the venom will continue to be pumped into the sting. Remove the stinger with an outward scraping motion of the fingernail. Do *not* pinch the stinger between two fingernails or grasp it with a tweezer, as these methods will force out more venom. Continue to scrape until it is free from the skin.
- Apply cold wet dressings to the sting; use ice if available.
- Relieve aching with one or two aspirin.
- For multiple stings or marked swelling, give the victim antihistamine tablets, if available.

STINGS BY SCORPIONS

Description: Scorpions are found in the United States from Louisiana to the southwestern states and in the desert and coastal regions of Mexico and Central America. Stings by these creatures are painful, and a few species inject a venom that is dangerous, even fatal to some children. Adults, however, almost always recover.

Symptoms include pain at the site of the bite, followed by numbness, weakness, and swelling in the surrounding area.

Treatment

- Apply cold wet dressings to the site of the scorpion sting.
- Have the victim rest.
- Then let the pain and swelling subside.
- A physician might administer antihistamines.
- If a child or infant is stung, get medical help.

STY

Description: A sty is an eyelid inflammation caused by the infection of the roots of the eyelashes or the oil glands. A small hard area appears on the edge of the eyelid, and soon a cyst filled with pus swells in the center of the infected area.

Often, the sty is a result of rubbing the eye with unclean hands.

Treatment

- *Be sure* the patient does not rub or touch the infected eyelid.
- Apply warm wet compresses to the affected area every two hours for about 15 minutes each time. After a few such treatments, the sty should open and the pus drain.
- Pat the area dry with a sterile gauze pad and let it remain open to the air.

NOTE: Many sties need to be lanced and should have a doctor's attention, especially if accompanied by signs of spreading infection, chills, or fever.

SECTION FIVE

An Ounce of Prevention

210

Tips that will help you prevent common medical emergencies before they happen.

Just about every severe injury to an adult can be prevented. It takes a state of mind that anticipates problems before they happen and one or more actions that remove the danger in time. Some people call this process "troubleshooting."

We all hurry too much, get careless from time to time, and get lost in our own thoughts, so that we are not alert to potential hazards.

These mistakes, and others, are even more apt to happen to children. They often don't know enough to avoid certain risks. Then, too, there are times when children and adults get excited and find themselves in situations they otherwise would have avoided.

Much of the following discussion presents commonsense advice. You may find it helpful to read for yourself and to use as instruction for your children.

AUTO SAFETY

Two thirds of all traffic accidents occur within twenty-five miles of home. Half of all fatal auto accidents occur at speeds *under* forty miles per hour and the driver is often under the influence of alcohol.

Almost *half* of all accidental deaths in the United States result from auto accidents.

We all believe such tragedies won't happen to us and those we love. Here's how to help make that belief a fact:

Keep Your Car in Top Mechanical Condition

- Read the owner's manual and follow the service instructions whether or not the car is still under warranty.
- At least once each week, take a good look at the tires to see if they're underinflated or overinflated. Also check the tire tread for excessive wear and for too much wear on one side or in the middle.
- At the same time, check the windshield wipers, the front and back lights, the brake lights, the directional signals, and the horn.
- Before going for a weekend trip or one that's longer, have a mechanic check your tires (including the spare), the steering system, brakes, brake fluid, hoses and belts, oil, transmission fluid, radiator, coolant, battery, exhaust system, windshield wipers, all lights, and wheel alignment.

Be in Good Condition Before You Drive

- Do not drive if you're overtired or have been drinking. Instead, put someone else behind the wheel, take a taxi or other public transportation, or stop and rest.
- Whenever you drive, keep passengers from distracting you.

Drive Defensively

- Wear seat belts and have your passengers wear them. Seat belts do save lives.
- Don't trust the other driver. Assume that he's careless, reckless, tired, or tipsy. Drive defensively.
- Give the car in front of you one car length for every ten miles per hour you're traveling.
- Use directional signals before changing lanes or making turns. But do *not* assume that others have seen your signals. Drive as if they have seen nothing, until their actions show that they are alert.
- Keep calm in heavy traffic. Accident risk increases with impatience.
- Speed limits save lives and fuel. Stay within them.
- Reduce your speed in rain and when visibility is poor.
- Keep your eyes on the driver ahead of you and the driver ahead of him. That way, you'll have advance warning of any need to brake, accelerate, or change lanes to avoid trouble.

Use Extra Precautions at Night

- In fact, you're safer if you drive at night only when necessary. The nighttime traffic death rate is two and one half times the daytime traffic death rate.
- When driving at night, decrease your daytime speed by at least 10 miles per hour.
- Be able to stop within your headlight range.
- Increase the space between you and the car in front.
- Turn your headlights on at dusk.

Be Prepared for an Emergency

- Carry the following items in your car at all times:
    1. Two pens.
    2. One pad of paper.
    3. Blanket.
    4. Fire extinguisher.

5. 2–6 flares or reflectors.
6. One flashlight with fresh batteries.
7. A record of your car insurance policy (not the policy itself).
8. A copy of your auto registration (unless state law requires you to carry the original).
9. Some change for phone calls.
10. A list of names, addresses, and phone numbers of your doctor and close relatives, in case you are found unconscious.

If You Have Car Trouble

- Pull as far off the road as possible.
- Place a flare or reflector 10 feet behind your car and another 200 feet behind your car. On a two-lane road, place a third flare or reflector 75 feet ahead of your vehicle.
- Leave on your emergency four-way flashers. (Caution: Women traveling alone at night may not want to call attention to car trouble. Many police departments recommend that women get the car off the road and put no lights on. Instead, wait for a police car to come by, then get the officers' attention. Or simply stay in the car all night until daybreak.)

BACK STRAIN

Back strain is not usually a critical injury, but a bad case of it can put a person in bed or cause major discomfort for several days. Most instances of back strain can be avoided.

Lift with Your Back Straight

- *Never* let the lower back arch forward as you lift any object, even one that's light.
- *Never* bend over stiff-legged to lift an object from the floor.
- Instead, place your feet close to the object, crouch with your back *straight,* feet flat on the floor or ground. Then grasp the object firmly and lift slowly using your *thigh* muscles. They are the strongest muscles in your body.

Don't Try to Lift If There's a Problem

- Do *not* lean over something, such as a radiator, to open a stuck window or to pick up an object. Get help instead. You and your partner should stand on the sides of whatever needs lifting.
- Do *not* keep trying to lift an object if you feel even a slight discomfort in your back.
- Do *not* reach to pick up something when one arm is loaded with other goods.

BITES BY ANIMALS

Most animal bites are made by pets that are *known* to the victim, not strange animals. The person has startled or somehow threatened the neighbor's, friend's, or even family's pet. Other animal bites are inflicted in self-defense. Very rarely is a bite made by a mad dog.

Avoid Teasing or Taunting Animals

- Whether the animal is a stray or a trusted friend, threatening him, getting him overly excited, or teasing him may cause him to bite.
- Keep away from any nervous animals.

Avoid Stray or Injured Animals

- Teach children to walk around strange dogs and cats, not to pat them, and not to pick them up.
- No adult or child should touch a badly injured animal, even if it's their own. Only specially trained personnel, who know how to avoid getting bitten, should touch an injured animal.

BURNS
(Also see FIRE, pg. 231.)

Burns and other emergencies caused by fire are the third-leading cause of accidental death. More than three quarters of deaths related to fires occur in the home.

Because children are victims in about 20 percent of fire fatalities, make sure the youngsters you love are familiar with the following information.

Teach Children That Hot Means Hurt

- Every young child should know enough to keep away from anything that's hot.
- Show each child that the following items can hurt them: matches, hot-water faucets, pots and pans on the stove, cigarettes, radiators, firescreens, electric heaters, furnaces, toasters, cigarette lighters, irons, candles, barbecue grills, and electric grills.

Keep Matches and Hot Cookware Out of Reach

- Hide matches or store them too high for youngsters to reach. Do *not* leave matches on counters and coffee tables. Remove cigarette lighters from the tops of tables too.
- Keep handles of pots and frying pans turned in on the kitchen range. Otherwise a child might tip them over, or you might hit them by accident, spilling hot liquids or foods.
- Do *not* put hot tea, coffee, or other liquids on a tablecloth that hangs way over the side of the table. Someone may trip on the cloth and spill scalding liquid.

- *Never* leave a small child alone in the bathtub. In addition to the danger of drowning, the youngster might turn on the hot-water faucet.
- While a child is in the bathtub, turn him so that he faces the hot-water faucet. That way, the youngster won't accidentally bump into the hot metal.
- *Never* leave children alone around an open fire, outdoor grill, fireplace, or glowing coals.
- Do *not* hold a child in your lap while you drink or pass hot beverages or while you smoke.

CUTS AND WOUNDS

There is no way to prevent all types of injury, but major cuts and wounds are most often avoidable.

Teach Children That Sharp Things Can Hurt

- Keep knives, scissors, razor blades, saws, saw blades, and all other sharp objects out of reach of small children.
- Teach children of all ages not to run with sharp objects in their hands or with lollipops or sticks in their mouths, and not to throw sharp objects.

Take Special Care When Using Sharp Tools and Guns

- Keep home-workshop tools disconnected. Lock switches and power supplies so children can't turn them on.
- Take care when using scissors, knives, or other sharp implements. When handing a knife to someone, always have the point turned *away* from him.
- *Always* keep firearms and ammunition locked in *separate* places. *Always* handle firearms with utmost caution.
- Be careful when handling power equipment. Plan ahead what you are going to do, and arrange that others do not distract you.

Clean up Broken Glass

- Keep your yard clean and free of broken glass, bottles, cans, boards, nails, and wire.
- If broken glass is found near places where children play, sweep it up promptly, even if it's not your glass or your area.

ELECTRIC SHOCKS

Electrical accidents can cause major burns and fatal shock.

Never Touch Electric Appliances with Wet Hands

- *Never* touch anything electrical while standing in water.
- *Never* place electric appliances where they can fall into any water.

Keep Electric Cords, Wires, and Outlets in Good Condition

- Replace frayed cords before they cause a burn or fire.
- Teach children not to play with electric cords, plugs, and outlets.
- Cover unused wall sockets with protective plastic plugs that will prevent children from pushing metal objects into the openings.
- Have electrical equipment permanently grounded.
- Before making electrical repairs, remove the fuse or throw the circuit breaker.
- Unless you have special training, it is best to let a repairman fix a malfunctioning appliance.
- Don't run extension cords under rugs; they wear easily and may short out, causing fire.

Always Avoid Fallen Wires

- *Never* touch a dangling wire. It may be charged by a crossed power line farther back. Report it to the utility company.
- If your car should run into a live wire, do *not* touch any metal. Stay in the car until help arrives. Rubber tires insulate car. If you must get out, *jump* out, do not touch the car while stepping to the ground.

EYE INJURIES

The eyes are among the most vulnerable parts of the body. Protect them by acting on the following information:

Keep Sharp Objects and Household Cleaners Away from Small Children

- Knives, scissors, needles, pincushions, and all sharp implements should be kept off tables, where they may fall or be taken by children.
- Adults and children should not run while carrying anything sharp.
- Keep small children away from BB guns, bows and arrows, darts, and other sharp or dangerous toys.
- Keep lye, cleaners, acids, and household chemicals closed tightly and stored out of reach of youngsters. Do *not* keep these chemicals under the kitchen or bathroom sink.

Be Careful While Using Tools

- Hobbyists and do-it-yourselfers should be cautious when using tools that can send metal or wood fragments flying.
- Wear protective goggles if the tools you use could cause sparks or objects to fly.

FALLS

(Also see Falls, pg. 65, for first aid.)

Falls kill and injure more people in the home than any other accident. Overall, falls are the second leading cause of accidental death. And studies show that most falls occur while people are walking on a horizontal surface.

Falls are the leading cause of accidental death and injury to people sixty-five years of age and older. Children, of course, have countless falls, but the more serious ones can be avoided by acting on these tips:

Remove Slipping and Tripping Hazards

- Wipe up spilled water, grease, and other liquids from the kitchen, bathroom, and garage floors as soon as possible.
- Clear away toys, shoes, tools, vacuum cleaner hoses, newspapers, and other items that can trip an unwary walker.
- Keep small footstools up against lounge chairs, where they are less likely to trip someone.
- *Never* store anything on stairs or stair landings. Find a safer storage area.
- Secure throw rugs with nonskid pads and keep them away from the top and bottom of stairs.
- Anchor rolled-up sections of carpets.
- Place a safety mat in the bathtub. Consider installing handholds, especially for an elderly person.
- Keep outside walks clear and clean. In winter, use salt or sand on icy areas.
- Beware of untied shoelaces.

Throw Some Light Where You're Walking

- Encourage the use of lights before entering a room, walking up or down stairs, and going down a corridor or hallway.
- Leave small lights on at night in the bathroom and, perhaps, in the hallways.
- Have family members use flashlights when they walk around late at night.

Use Caution When Climbing, Reaching, and Carrying

- Do *not* use chairs or boxes for climbing. Instead, be safe with a sturdy stepladder.
- Check the rungs on ladders before use. Position the ladder securely before climbing. When up the ladder, do not overreach. Climb down the ladder instead, and reposition it.
- Periodically inspect steps, handrails, and stair carpets to make sure they are in good condition. If not, make repairs immediately. Carpeted stairways, for example, should be tacked securely at the base of each riser and at the top and bottom.
- If your basement stairs are to be painted, add a little sand to the paint for a better grip. Or install rubber or abrasive treads.
- Do *not* overload yourself by carrying objects that are too heavy or block your vision. Get assistance.

POISONING BY INHALATION

Preventing poisoning by inhalation is simple:

Use Poisonous Substances Only in Well-ventilated Areas

- *Never* start a car in a closed garage. *Always* open the doors before turning on the ignition, even if it's cold outside.
- Use poisonous sprays inside only when several windows are open and there is a draft of fresh air.
- Wear a mask over your mouth and nose when spraying paints, pesticides, and similar toxic substances. This will prevent inhaling harmful particles. Plenty of ventilation is needed for toxic fumes.
- *Never* light a barbecue fire in an enclosed area. Light such fires outside in appropriate areas or in an interior fireplace.

POISONING BY MOUTH

Your home is full of poisons. Medications that will help a person will harm *anyone* if taken to excess. Soaps, cleaners, waxes, food extracts, gasoline, cosmetics, and other common substances are potentially fatal if swallowed.

Over one half million youngsters are poisoned in their homes each year. Preschoolers are the most likely victims.

Use Child-proof Containers Correctly

- If there are children in your home, always ask that prescriptions be filled in child-proof containers. Open and close these bottles in the way that can prevent a child from doing the same. Don't defeat the container's purpose.

Keep Medications, Cleaners, and Other Poisons Out of Children's Reach

- Store rubbing alcohol and other toxic liquids as high up as possible.
- Because toddlers and children climb and are likely to explore the medicine cabinet, keep harmful substances in child-proof containers or locked away elsewhere.
- Do *not* leave laundry soaps, disinfectants, detergents, bleach, toilet-bowl cleaners, and similar items under sinks or on top of washing machines. Lock them away or store them high up and out of sight.
- Do *not* leave gasoline, kerosene, lighter fluid, and similar poisons in the garage where children can find them.
- Always place insect and rodent poisons in out-of-the-way storage areas, and lock them up.

- Even cosmetics—such as hair sprays, nail polish, nail-polish remover, cologne, and similar preparations—are dangerous if swallowed. Store them carefully.
- Keep youngsters from gnawing on surfaces that have been finished with lead paint. Select toys with lead-free paint.

Teach Children That Poisons Are Like Fire: They Hurt

- As soon as children are old enough to understand, point out the drugs, chemicals, and other substances to be avoided.

Be Careful When Taking Medications

- *Never* take medications in the dark.
- Don't store sleeping pills in night tables. Such a convenience can cause an accidental overdose.
- *Always* read the label before taking any drug. Keep all bottles clearly labeled.
- Dispose of any old or unused drugs promptly by flushing them down the toilet.

RESPIRATORY FAILURE

Drowning accidents are the fourth leading cause of accidental death. In addition to drowning and drownproofing, choking, suffocation, and strangulation are the subjects of the following discussion.

DROWNING

Prevent this tragedy by observing these rules:

Everyone Should Know How to Swim

- All children aged about three and older should know how to swim.
- Do *not* overestimate your ability to swim long distance.
- Do *not* overextend yourself while swimming underwater. If, while underwater, your chest feels tight and you need air, come directly to the surface.

Know and Observe Water Safety Rules

- *Never* leave a baby or small child alone in a bathtub or wading pool.
- Swimming pools, wading pools, and fishponds should be surrounded by sturdy fences and swinging gates that have safety locks.
- *Never* swim alone. No matter how accomplished a swimmer you are, always swim where there are lifeguards or with a friend.
- Beware of unfamiliar swimming areas. Before entering them, know about currents, deep holes, debris, rocks, and other hazards. And never dive into unfamiliar water. *Be sure* to find out all about rocks and shallow areas first.

- Do not swim immediately after eating or when overheated or tired.
- Do not swim after drinking alcoholic beverages.
- Stop swimming when you become tired or cold.
- *Never* dunk anyone or hold a person's head underwater.
- *Never* push anyone into the water.
- Make sure that young children wear life jackets when playing in or even near pools and other water.

Practice Drownproofing Techniques

- Rest underwater. Be as relaxed as possible.
- Then move your body up slightly so your nostrils extend above the water.
- Exhale hard through your *nose* just as it rises into the air. Exhale through the nose (not the mouth) so your nostrils retain no water to drip down your throat. Keep your lips sealed tightly. Then raise your head above water.
- Inhale with your *mouth.*
- Then relax, and let yourself sink below the surface.
- When submerged, spit out any water you have retained.
- Stay submerged a minimum of 3 seconds at a time before repeating the procedure. Gradually increase the time submerged to 10 seconds.
- After practicing this drownproofing method, you can remain in the water for several hours without becoming exhausted.

CHOKING

Ordinary objects such as food and pieces of toys often cause choking.

Be Aware of the Insignificant Objects That Can Choke a Small Child

- Check all toys to *be sure* eyes, nose, knobs, and other parts will not come off when pulled or chewed.

- Until age four, do *not* give children nuts, candies containing nuts, uncooked vegetables, fruits that require chewing, uncooked meat, or any foods containing hard seeds or pits.
- Similarly, do *not* allow a small child to play with beans, peas, corn kernels, seeds, or other small but hard foods.
- Keep coins, bottle caps, buttons, pins, tacks, and similar objects out of the reach of small children.
- Inspect meat, fish, and poultry for bones and shells before serving.
- Do not permit a child to run while eating.
- Discourage laughing while food is in the mouth.
- As soon as possible, discourage children from putting foreign objects in their mouths.

Chew Food Slowly and Carefully

- Cut food into small pieces before putting anything in your mouth. Be alert for seeds, shells, and small pieces of bone.
- If you wear dentures, keep them in good repair.
- *Never* sleep with anything in your mouth.
- If something is lodged in your throat, remain calm. Wait until the spasm passes, then cough hard to expel the foreign body.
- If diners are drinking alcohol with the meal or if they are elderly, be alert for the chance that some part of the meal might lodge temporarily in the throat.

SUFFOCATION AND STRANGULATION

Suffocation and strangulation are the leading cause of accidental death to infants under one year old. Accidental strangulation also occurs to older children and adults.

Be Aware That Ordinary Objects Can Suffocate or Strangle

- *Never* place a plastic bag or thin plastic covering near an infant or small child. Do *not* cover the crib with this material. Thin plastic can block the mouth and nose and lead to asphyxiation.
- Do *not* place a pillow in a crib, because it can cause suffocation.
- Do *not* allow youngsters of any age to play with string, venetian-blind cords, rope, jewelry, or wires that can wind around their necks.
- Do *not* place an infant's crib where it can come into contact with the cord of a venetian blind.

SECTION SIX

Fire Safety

Prevention, Escape, and Control

Each year in the United States, twelve thousand people die in fires, and another three hundred thousand are badly burned.

Most of the fatalities are not the result of burns. They are caused by smoke inhalation. Many people die in their sleep, overcome by the deadly gases.

This section discusses how to to react and how not to react when a fire occurs in your home, how to develop and carry through a fire-escape plan, and how to prevent home fires.

Reacting to a Fire

Three elements are needed to cause and maintain any fire:

1. Fuel (paper, clothes, rags, grease, wood, etc.).
2. Heat (from a match, cigarette, faulty electrical wires, etc.).
3. Air.

Small Fires

- Even if the fire is confined to a frying pan or a wastebasket, it is safest to yell, "Fire!" and tell everyone to get out of the home. Evacuate everyone first.
- Then take 30 seconds to fight the fire. But small fires can grow with frightening speed. *Never* risk your life or anyone else's. *Leave after 30 seconds.*

For Wood, Paper, and Fabric Fires

- Eliminate the fuel by carrying it or throwing it out of the home.
- Or cut off the air. Smother the fire with a rug, coat, or heavy woolen blanket.

- Or eliminate the heat. Cool the fire with water, a fire extinguisher, sand, or earth.

Remember: *Leave after 30 seconds.*

For Electrical Fires

- Shut off the electricity.
- Then extinguish the flames with water, sand, or earth.
- Or smother them with a rug, coat, or blanket.
- But if you can't shut off the electricity, *never* use water. That will splatter the flames. Instead, use a Class C fire extinguisher (for more information on extinguishers, see pg. 237).

Remember: *Leave after 30 seconds.*

For Oil or Grease Fires

- Eliminate the air by covering a flaming pan with a lid. Or smother the flames with sand, earth, a rug, or a blanket.
- Or use a Class B fire extinguisher.
- *Never* use water on an oil or grease fire, for that will splatter the flames.

Remember: *Leave after 30 seconds.*

For a Gas Fire

- Shut off the gas.
- Then cool the fire with water, sand, or earth.
- Or smother it with a blanket.
- If you can't shut off the gas, *get out.*

After extinguishing a small fire, it is safest to call the fire department and tell them what happened. They may suggest ways to be sure the fire is out, or they may want to inspect it themselves.

Remember: *Leave after 30 seconds.*

Large Fires

- Alert all others. If at home, yell, "Fire!" (in a crowded place it may be best to quietly inform people of a fire, so that they remain calm). It may or may not be possible to knock on doors, check rooms, or talk with others. So once you know a fire has broken out, yell that fact *loudly.*
- *Get out.* Every room in your home should have at least two escape routes (discussed below). You are responsible for getting yourself out. You can never be sure you'll be able to get others out too. (Also discussed below is an escape plan to help ensure that children get themselves out.)
- Congregate. All members of your family or other people you live with should meet at a *predetermined* point outside the home. That's the only sure way of knowing that everyone has escaped.
- Notify the fire department. It's best for an adult to put in the call by pulling an alarm, phoning from a neighbor's, dialing 911, or calling the operator. Do *not* assume that someone else has contacted the fire department. It's much better for them to get several calls than none. *You* make sure they know about it.
- *Never* re-enter a burning house. Not for a pet, a mink stole, jewelry, cash, items of sentimental value. Nothing. Otherwise there's a good chance you'll have to be carried out.

FIRE PLAN

The five points listed are the main objectives for any fire plan. Briefly, they are:

1. Alert all others.
2. Get out.
3. Congregate.
4. Notify the fire department.
5. Never re-enter a burning building.

It is vital to the safety of all who live with you that everyone participate in the development of a fire plan. Fire is a terrifying experience, but thorough familiarity with a fire plan will give you and your family an alternative to panic.

Everyone will know what to do and will be more likely to do it.

How to Make a Fire Plan

- Make a floor plan of your house or apartment. Label all rooms. Indicate all doors, windows, stairways, fire escapes, porches, roofs, and roofs of nearby buildings.
- Mark two escape routes for each room in your home. This is especially vital for bedrooms. Most home fires occur at night when the occupants are asleep.
- The first escape route from a bedroom should show the simplest way to the ground (opening a window and climbing out, for example, if appropriate).
- The second escape route from a bedroom should show an emergency path, in case the normal route is impassable (if, for example, the fire is near the windows, note the halls and stairways to take to safety).
- *Never* obstruct the opening of all windows in a bedroom. If you have keyed locks or wrought-iron grills, for example, *make sure* at

least one bedroom window is free of them and easy to open all the way.

- *Never* obstruct access to a fire escape by placing a keyed lock or an accordion gate at the access window.
- If any window in the home might not open easily, make sure everyone knows that it's all right to break it with a chair, shoe, lamp, or other hard object.
- Instruct everyone to break the window wide enough so that no jagged pieces can harm him or her.
- Then he or she must throw a blanket over the windowsill to further avoid getting cut.
- Seriously consider always sleeping with bedroom doors closed. The bedroom door can be the best protection against fire, smoke, gases, and superheated air. The closed door can save your life and the lives of your children. If everyone knows how to get out the safest way, there may be no need to go and see if the children are all right. Shouting to them will reassure them and guide them to safety.
- Be sure to use porches, roofs, and other structures to alert neighbors.
- If appropriate, use a rope ladder or an aluminum ladder attached to the roof or the inside sill of an upstairs window. In some cases, the ladder is the best escape route.
- Make sure everyone knows the following facts about fire:
  1. The hot air and poisonous gases rise, so it is usually safer to *stay close to the floor,* perhaps even crawling to an exit.
  2. When getting out of bed during a fire, do *not* stand up. Instead, roll out of bed onto the floor to take advantage of the cooler, safer air.
  3. Before opening a bedroom door from the inside, feel the wood and doorknob. If they are hot, leave the door closed. Fire is on the other side!
  4. If you decide to open a bedroom door from the inside, do so slowly with your foot braced against it. That way, you'll be better prepared to shut the door fast against the great force of superheated air.
  5. Rather than run down a smoky or fire-filled hall, it's often safer to *remain behind a closed door* and wait for help. Stuff cloths, blankets, or other soft materials at the bottom of the door to help keep out smoke and gases.

6. If your clothing catches on fire, *do not run,* because that will fan the flames. Instead, lie down with your hands covering your face and roll back and forth slowly to smother the fire. Or someone can smother the flames by wrapping a heavy coat, scatter rug, or blanket around you.

- Agree upon a place outside the home where everyone must meet.
- After everyone has assembled, decide who is to call the fire department. *When calling the fire department* (or 911 or "0"), clearly state:
  1. Where you live (city or town, street number, and street name).
  2. That there's a fire, and tell them how large.
  3. Your name.
  4. Then wait for any questions they might have.
- If there are children in your home, appoint one or more of the older children to be "fire bosses." Their job will be to help evacuate the youngsters.
- Practice your fire plan at least once each month with a surprise fire drill. Make sure everyone who opens a closed door tests it first.

Smoke Detectors and Fire Extinguishers

You will want to at least consider installing one or more smoke detectors as well as one or more fire extinguishers.

Smoke Detectors

Smoke detectors are far more effective early-warning devices than are heat detectors or flame detectors. Only smoke detectors are designed to discern the visible and invisible combustion particles and smoke, then sound an alarm when these poisonous gases reach a predetermined level. *Remember* that most home-fire deaths are caused by inhalation of poisonous gases.

- Some detectors are available as single units for about twenty dollars.
- Or as complete systems, which consist of several units connected to a common alarm that rings in one or more rooms of the home. The complete systems sometimes are connected to the local fire department, too. Systems start at around five hundred dollars.

- The two basic types of smoke detectors are the optical (also called photoelectric) and the ionization chamber. Either type is fine for home use.
- Take a look at your fire plan to determine the best placement of one or more smoke detection units or the placement of units within a complete system. Smoke detectors should be situated near the bedrooms, so that smoke from a fire originating in another area must pass by the early-warning unit before reaching people who are asleep.
- Seriously consider adding smoke detectors in bedrooms that are occupied by people who smoke at night, as well as elderly, bedridden, or handicapped persons.
- All units or systems should be approved by a recognized testing laboratory such as Underwriters' Laboratories (UL), Underwriters' Laboratories of Canada (ULC), or Factory Mutual System (FM).

Fire Extinguishers

- Fire extinguishers should be approved by one of the same laboratories, UL, ULC, or FM.
- Fire extinguishers are to be used *only* to put out *small fires* in a wastebasket or frying pan, for example, or to help fight your way to *safety.* Home fire extinguishers are too small to accomplish any but those two objectives.
- So use this equipment only for *30 seconds* to fight a small fire and get out, or to help you move directly to safety.
- Whenever you use a fire extinguisher, yell, "Fire!" to others in the home. Have them get to safety immediately.

Class A Extinguishers—Small Wood, Paper, and Fabric Fires

- Water from a hose or glass is the best extinguisher for these common fires (but *not* for flammable liquid or electrical fires). Consider placing hoses under all bathroom sinks, with enough hose to reach the length of all rooms on the floor, and in the kitchen. A simple attachment lets you slip one end of the hose over the faucet.
- A Class A fire extinguisher (for wood, paper, or fabric) does the same work as water, plus it usually will have fire-retardant additives.

Class A fires are the most common in the home, but because water combats them as well as these units, Class A fire extinguishers are not the most popular. They usually cost under ten dollars.

Class B Extinguishers—Small Flammable-Liquid Fires

- Class B fire extinguishers (for flammable liquids such as grease, oil, gasoline, and other petroleum products and chemicals) are good for use in the kitchen, garage, and workshop.

Class C Extinguishers—Small Electrical Fires

- Class C fire extinguishers (for electrical fires) are good for use in the kitchen and the laundry room.

Other Fire Extinguishers

Combination Class B and Class C fire extinguishers are available as B:C extinguishers. They are the most popular, because they do everything that water cannot.

Some stores also carry combination A:B:C fire extinguishers, which are good for virtually all home fires. Their cost is about twenty dollars or more.

NOTE: After you have used your fire extinguisher, no matter how small the fire, give the fire department a call on their non-emergency line. Tell these experts what happened, how you responded, and the present status of the fire. Then let them tell you what, if anything, to do next.

PREVENTION

Most fires in the home result from carelessness. We don't think about some things—and don't want to think about others—but a fire can happen in your house or apartment. That's why almost everyone has fire insurance.

But no insurance really pays for the suffering caused by burns or the grief caused by a fire-related death.

Take the time *now* to check your home and prevent a fire:

- *Be aware* of the habits of any smoker in your home. If someone who lives with you smokes regularly, or if guests smoke, insist that they always use ashtrays—not wastebaskets—for their ashes; that they never leave lit cigarettes unattended on the lips of ashtrays; and that they never smoke in bed or while lounging in an easy chair.
- *Never* leave matches and cigarette lighters where children can reach them. Instead, keep them high up and hidden away. Teach children that matches, cigarette lighters, and the stove can *hurt* them.
- Do *not* leave young children unattended.
- *Be sure* that baby-sitters know and follow your safety rules.
- Protect sources of heat from flammables. Have a screen in front of your fireplace. Be careful that clothes and curtains can't blow into or even near electric heaters, stoves, fireplaces, and other heat sources. Do not place any flammables (such as papers or magazines) near furnaces, stoves, and the like.
- Fire hazards include messy and junk-filled attics, basements, garages, and closets. Clean them out regularly.
- Immediately dispose of oily rags or keep them tightly covered in a metal can. Otherwise they can cause a fire by themselves.
- Immediately replace all frayed electric cords.
- Use extension cords sparingly. And temporarily, not permanently. Do *not* run extension cords under a rug.

- Do *not* connect too many appliances and fixtures to any one circuit. If you do, hot wires within your walls will result, possibly causing a fire. Signs of hot wires are fuses that blow frequently, toasters and coffee brewers that heat slowly, television sets with pictures that flicker or shrink, and radios whose output fades or sounds scratchy. If these signs occur, call an electrician. Only experienced people should check and, if necessary, replace faulty wiring.
- If your heating plant is cracked, the pipes are rusty, or the chimney is clogged, have them examined immediately.
- Have a heating contractor inspect your heating system at least once each year. The best time is before winter.
- If you suspect a gas leak, call the gas company or a heating contractor immediately. Then open doors and windows, and get yourself and all others out until the technician arrives.
- Be sure to follow the manufacturer's instructions when installing and using petroleum-burning heaters. Repair or replace defective parts.
- Chimneys and wood stoves should be cleaned and inspected often—depending on how much they are used.
- *Never* store or leave gasoline in the home. It is highly volatile.
- *Never* store or leave benzine or naphtha in the home. They, too, are highly flammable.
- Never use gasoline, benzine, or naphtha as cleaning agents, because of their flammability.

INDEX

A

B

C

D

E

F

G

H

I

J

K

L

M

N

O

P

R

S

T

U

V

W

Y

EMERGENCY PHONE NUMBERS

	ADDRESS	
FIRE DEPT.		PHONE
POLICE (LOCAL)	ADDRESS	PHONE
POLICE (STATE)	ADDRESS	PHONE

REMEMBER: If you can't reach a doctor, dial 0 for Operator. Tell the operator you have an emergency and give the correct address. The operator will assist you in obtaining medical attention.

	ADDRESSES	
DOCTOR		PHONE
AMBULANCE		PHONE
PARAMEDICS		PHONE
HOSPITAL		PHONE
CARDIAC UNIT		PHONE
POISON CONTROL CENTER		PHONE
PHARMACY		PHONE
TAXICAB		PHONE
RELATIVE		PHONE
NEIGHBOR		PHONE